DOCTORS IN DISPUTE

Dr Lee Forrester is determined to overcome Dr Grant Sinclair's unreasoning prejudice against women when she arrives, newly qualified, to work as locum in her uncle's general practice. For the younger partner's hostile arrogance is almost medieval...

*Books you will enjoy
in our Doctor–Nurse series*

FLYAWAY SISTER by Lisa Cooper
TROPICAL NURSE by Margaret Barker
LADY IN HARLEY STREET by Anne Vinton
FIRST-YEAR'S FANCY by Lynne Collins
DESERT FLOWER by Dana James
INDIAN OCEAN DOCTORS by Juliet Shore
CRUISE NURSE by Clare Lavenham
CAPTIVE HEART by Hazel Fisher
A PROFESSIONAL SECRET by Kate Norway
NURSE ON CALL by Leonie Craig
THE GILDED CAGE by Sarah Franklin
A SURGEON CALLED AMANDA by Elizabeth Harrison
VICTORY FOR VICTORIA by Betty Neels
SHAMROCK NURSE by Elspeth O'Brien
ICE VENTURE NURSE by Lydia Balmain
TREAD SOFTLY, NURSE by Lynne Collins
DR VENABLES' PRACTICE by Anne Vinton
NURSE OVERBOARD by Meg Wisgate
EMERGENCY NURSE by Grace Read
WRONG DOCTOR JOHN by Kate Starr

DOCTORS IN DISPUTE

BY
JEAN EVANS

MILLS & BOON LIMITED
London · Sydney · Toronto

*First published in Great Britain 1983
by Mills & Boon Limited, 15–16 Brook's Mews,
London W1A 1DR*

© Jean Evans 1983

*Australian copyright 1983
Philippine copyright 1983*

ISBN 0 263 74380 2

All the characters in this book have no existence outside the imagination of the Author, and have no relation whatsoever to anyone bearing the same name or names. They are not even distantly inspired by any individual known or unknown to the Author, and all the incidents are pure invention.

The text of this publication or any part thereof may not be reproduced or transmitted in any form or by any means, electronic or mechanical, including photocopying, recording, storage in an information retrieval system, or otherwise, without the written permission of the publisher.

This book is sold subject to the condition that it shall not, by way of trade or otherwise, be lent, resold, hired out or otherwise circulated without the prior consent of the publisher in any form of binding or cover other than that in which it is published and without a similar condition including this condition being imposed on the subsequent purchaser.

Set in 11 on 12½ pt Linotron Times
03/0883

*Photoset by Rowland Phototypesetting Ltd
Bury St Edmunds, Suffolk
Made and printed in Great Britain by
Richard Clay (The Chaucer Press) Ltd
Bungay, Suffolk*

CHAPTER ONE

LEE FORRESTER edged the car out of the mainstream of traffic into a lay-by and switched off the engine. Hunting in the glove compartment she drew out a map, unfolded it and, having poured a cup of coffee from the thermos on the seat beside her, began studying the criss-cross of lines which would eventually bring her to the village of Foxley.

Her finger traced the route and a glance at her watch showed almost one o'clock. She had made good time despite the sudden downpour and a stop for a cup of tea just north of Oxford. With a bit of luck she should make her destination easily by four.

Draining the coffee she flicked the dregs out of the window, screwed the top back on the thermos and freshened up quickly with a tissue, using the vanity mirror to flick a comb through her hair. The reflection which stared back at her showed a small, oval face framed by a cap of short, blonde hair which turned rebelliously up at the ends despite all attempts to quell it, making her look ridiculously younger than her twenty-five years. It had been the cause of a lot of teasing at Medical School where she had been labelled the infant of the group. Not that she had minded. It had all been good natured teasing, but a frown momentarily etched its way into her forehead. She could see that it might become a problem. Her delicate bone structure was emphasised by large, blue eyes and a mouth which smiled slightly as her glance fell upon the letter in her open bag. She knew the words by heart but a tiny tremor of excitement still ran through her as she read it again. *'Dear Dr Forrester...'* Doctor. It was going to take some time to get used to the idea that she had actually passed her final exams and earned the title for which she had struggled for so long.

Popping the letter into her bag she re-started the car and eased back into the traffic, her mind still caught up in the memory of those years of dedicated training at a large teaching hospital in the South. Looking back on it now it was all a bit like a dream. Had there really been times when she had almost given it all up? It was surprising how easily one forgot the numbing tiredness which came after days of lectures combined with the more practical business of surgeons' rounds when, as medical students, a crowd of young hopefuls had followed the great man, Sir Horace Flinders, through the wards. There had been times, she had to admit, when the final goal had seemed an eternity away and only the knowledge that she wasn't alone in those feelings had kept her going. But now it was worth it and she was actually about to take up her first post, even if it had come about in a rather unorthodox manner.

It was raining again and she set the windscreen

wipers in motion, hoping it wasn't going to snow. It had been a long winter and a promise of spring had proved to be tantalisingly brief. Still, it couldn't last for ever. Another week and it would be April. The reminder had come from her father when he had first broached the subject of the job to her and she had jokingly responded that the Midlands in the depths of winter weren't the ideal place to be.

John Forrester had viewed his daughter with a twinkle in his eye as he made a stabbing motion in her direction with his pipe.

'You're just plain scared, my girl. Looking for an excuse to avoid taking up your responsibilities. Well, you won't be able to do it for ever, you know. You've worked hard for that qualification and it's time you started putting it to good use.'

Her laughter had faded as she looked at him, the wide eyes suddenly serious. 'Oh Dad, it's not that, it's just . . . well, I'm scared. I know it's stupid and I'm ashamed to admit it, but now that the crunch has come I'm scared out of my wits.'

Contrary to her expectations her father hadn't laughed. Instead he had settled back in his chair, looked around the modest but well used surgery and frowned. 'I know the feeling and in spite of what you may be thinking you aren't alone. If it's any consolation I felt exactly the same thirty years ago when I qualified and came here.'

'You did?' She stared at him incredulously, unaware of how alike they were, not only in temperament but in looks too at that moment, even though there were now flecks of grey in her father's hair. 'I find it hard to imagine.'

'I know, but it's true, and if any doctor tells you he isn't scared, then I can only guess he's lying. It's not an easy profession you've chosen, my dear. The work is hard, often unrewarding, and the responsibilities increase as patients get to know you and put their faith in you and your judgments. There will be times when you'll be wrong. Pray God, rarely, but it can happen. We're fallible, Lee, human, and we don't have all the answers, and even if we do the answer isn't always in our hands. But sooner or later you've got to take the first step, decide whether all those years of training were for something or not.'

She studied him, feeling a new sense of calm growing inside her. 'It's what I've always wanted, you know that.'

He laughed. 'I should. I taught you to bandage your dolls and I lost count of the times you knocked at this door begging me to take their temperatures.'

It was funny, but she had forgotten it until he reminded her. 'Well, I guess it's not dolls any more, is it? This is for real and you're right, I've got to start somewhere.'

'You don't want to go on and specialise?'

She shook her head, quite definite about that. 'No. I like the idea of getting to know a community, of working and living with them. The formality of a hospital doesn't appeal.'

He nodded. 'I felt the same way and I've never

regretted the decision to become a GP. I'm only sorry there isn't scope for a partner here. You know there's nothing I'd like better than to have you with me.'

'I know, and there's nothing I'd like better than to be here.' She reached out to press a hand on his arm. 'But it's probably as well that I start somewhere else and learn to stand on my own feet.'

'Have you anywhere specific in mind?'

'No.' She frowned, brushing her hair back in a gesture he recognised well. 'I suppose I've been putting it off. I've made some enquiries, of course, but nothing definite has come of it.'

John Forrester took the pipe from his mouth and foraged on the desk for a letter which he handed to her. 'Read that. In a way it might be the hand of providence.' He sat in silence as she scanned the single page, then her glance flew up to meet him.

'Oh Dad, I can't believe it. Not Uncle Tom. Why didn't you tell me?'

He shrugged. 'You had other problems on your mind. Apparently the heart attack happened a couple of months ago, his partner wrote to tell me.'

'Is it very bad?'

'According to young Sinclair it would have been enough to finish anyone less determined.'

Her face paled and she studied the letter again. 'Sinclair?'

'Grant Sinclair. Tom's partner. We've corresponded a couple of times since he wrote telling me what had happened. He's been keeping me up to date on his progress but I can guess for myself that Tom must be feeling a lot better if he managed to write that.'

The handwriting was less firm than she remembered but still recognisable and she found herself wondering vaguely why the medical profession were always notorious for their barely legible scrawl. 'He says he isn't going to be back at work for at least another three months and then only on light duties, which presumably means no night or emergency calls.'

'That's why he wrote.' He gestured towards the page. 'He says it's a growing practice and that although Grant has taken over the entire load until now, it's obviously more than one man can handle alone and he's going to have to get a locum in.' There was a moment's silence during which she thought she sensed what was coming and was proved right when he said simply. 'How about it, Lee?'

She laughed, awkwardly. 'But I don't know anything about this . . . Grant Sinclair, Dad.'

'Does that matter. You know Tom.'

'Yes, of course. He's always been just like a real uncle to me, you know that, and I'd like to help. In a way I almost feel I owe it, after all it was Tom Jameson who first put the idea of medicine into my head.' She wrinkled her nose. 'More relevant really is the fact that this Grant Sinclair doesn't know me. How do you imagine he's likely to take to the idea of having a newly qualified doctor as his locum?'

Her father applied a match to his pipe and puffed in silence for a moment, looking at her through a haze of smoke. 'Why not write and ask him?' There was almost a hint of challenge in his eyes. 'This could be the somewhere you have to start, my dear, and if it will help old Tom, you'd be doing me a favour as well.'

She opened her mouth and closed it again, but that night she wrote the letter, briefly outlining her qualifications and the fact that she had trained at St Clements. She posted it next morning and promptly dismissed it from her mind so that when, a few days later, a reply plopped through the letter box just as she was going in to breakfast she had to fight a sudden feeling of unreasoned panic.

Sitting at the table she read the reply. It was brief almost to the point of being curt. It said simply, 'Dear Dr Forrester, having spoken with Dr Jameson, who assures me that he has every faith in your ability to undertake the post, I shall look forward to seeing you one week from today. I should take this opportunity to warn you, however, that, whilst Foxley is a village, we are a growing community and also take patients from the surrounding areas, so that you must be prepared to work whatever hours are considered necessary.'

It was signed 'Yours sincerely, Grant Sinclair.'

Reading the letter through again she decided that he sounded thoroughly pompous and that he certainly wasn't going to be easy to work with, but as it was only for three months she could stick it, if only to repay her father and old Tom Jameson in some small measure for all they had done for her over the years.

Resolution faltered just a little, however, as the blue Mini ate up the miles bringing her closer to Foxley. She sped easily enough through Market Harborough and into Kibworth Beauchamp where she pulled in upon a spur of the moment decision to take lunch at a charming pub called the Coach and Horses. Three centures old, the atmosphere was warm and friendly and the food excellent. It was only as she sat before a roaring fire, tucking into a delicious home-made steak and kidney pie that she realised just how hungry she was, which probably accounted for the nervous fluttering in her stomach she chided herself. But it was banished by the superb meal and a cup of coffee and she set off again feeling rather more than comfortably full but ready for anything—even Grant Sinclair.

The rain unfortunately gave way to the first flakes of snow as she drove round Leicester and into the open countryside where it was hard to imagine that the ground would be carpeted by millions of bluebells in a few weeks. Promising herself a visit to Bradgate, home of the ill-fated Lady Jane Grey, she spotted the turning for Foxley, estimating after another brief look at the map that it must be about five miles away.

The streets were busy with shoppers so that when she saw the small crowd gathered she wasn't at first concerned. It was only as she glanced towards it and glimpsed the figure lying in the road that she realised there had been an accident and someone was obviously hurt. A young woman was weeping distractedly and Lee felt a momentary rush of anger as she saw the crowd press in, morbid curiosity on their faces. 'And I'll bet no one has thought to call an ambulance,' she thought, grimly, as she brought the car to a halt. Her initial instinct not to get involved disappeared as she got out and saw the blood spattered over the man's clothing. Someone was trying to lift him and, swinging the car door open, she got out, and hurried towards the spot, saying sharply, 'Don't do that. Don't make any attempt to move him. Can't you see he's hurt and unconscious?'

The woman stared at her, muttered something and moved aside as Lee knelt swiftly, her fingers already feeling for a pulse. She breathed a sigh of relief. At least he was alive though he was pale and was losing blood at an alarming rate.

'I'm a doctor,' she explained quickly, sensing a tiny flicker of resentment. 'Has someone called an ambulance?'

The mood of the crowd changed to one of instant relief. 'I'll see to it, Doctor. Good job you came along.' Someone sprinted away, she didn't look up to see who, her attention was on the man who moaned softly as he came round and stared up at her with understandable confusion.

'What . . . what the devil happened?'

'Please lie quite still, just while I check you over,'

she advised, smiling gently. 'An ambulance is on its way.'

He brushed a hand against his head, making contact with the blood. She was able to reassure him, having made a cursory examination which to her relief showed it to be nothing more serious than a cut, albeit a fairly deep one, caused when he had stepped off the kerb and slipped on the icy road surface, bumping his head. The wound was probably going to need a few stitches but it wouldn't leave a scar. She studied him more closely as she looked with rather more concern at the gash in his arm and began applying a tourniquet made out of her own clean handkerchief. He was about thirty she judged and probably quite good-looking under different circumstances.

She shivered, wishing the ambulance would get a move on. It was still snowing and the man's pallor indicated that he was suffering from shock as much as from the cold. It was disconcerting to look down and find him studying her with equal intensity.

His mouth formed a crooked smile. 'Sorry, I don't even know your name to thank you. This must be a damned nuisance.'

'Not at all.' She smiled quickly. 'I'm just glad I happened to be around. I expect the ambulance will be along soon.'

She wondered briefly what time it was. The light was already fading and she still had to find her exact destination. The man winced as he tried to move.

'I haven't seen you around these parts before. You must be a stranger.'

'Why?' Her lips curved. 'Do you know everyone?'

'Most. There's not much goes on in a small community that the locals don't get to know about, you know. Are you staying or passing through?'

She laughed. 'That rather depends on how far it is to Foxley.' She caught the quick flicker of interest in his eyes as she bent to check the tourniquet, then suddenly a voice came angrily from behind her and a hand jerked her roughly to her feet.

'For God's sake, don't you know better than to practise amateurish first aid when you don't have a clue what you're doing?'

Colour flooded angrily into her cheeks as she found herself staring into a pair of steely-grey eyes set in a face which was taut with accusation as the man faced her. Her gaze briefly took in a square jaw and dark hair, dampened by snow. It would have been a handsome face except for the arrogance which darkened the chiselled features as he stared past her and thrust her painfully aside as he knelt beside the man who had mercifully lapsed into unconsciousness again.

His gaze was thrust upwards as he stared at her, taking in the small, pale oval of her face. She looked like a child with her blonde hair plastered down by the snow.

'I just hope you haven't done any real damage,' his voice was cold with fury, 'because if so, you'd better be prepared to face the consequences. Now get out of my way.'

Without giving her a chance to speak he turned away, leaving her standing, shaking with angry resentment while the crowd moved in, sensing some additional drama. Her mouth opened briefly upon a sharp retort that she was a doctor and knew perfectly well what she was doing, then in the distance she heard the siren of the approaching ambulance and, tight-lipped, she stepped back, blinking hard to stop the tears which pricked at her eyes. The injustice of the attack stayed with her even as she walked back to her car, got in and drove away as quickly as possible from the scene and the memory of the man who had taken charge, dismissing her as if she were an incompetent schoolgirl. How dare he? Her hands tightened against the steering wheel.

She was still trembling when she drove into the village and finally located Tom Jameson's house. She sat for a moment trying to regather her composure before knocking on the door to meet the man with whom she would be working. One bad-tempered individual in a day was quite enough, she thought. Then her ill humour vanished as she climbed the front steps and moments later found herself enveloped in an embrace by her father's dearest friend and before she knew it they were sitting before the warmth of a fire, exchanging news and laughter over a cup of tea.

'I can't tell you how delighted I am to have you

here.' Tom Jameson sat in his comfortable arm chair studying her. 'I've watched your progress, from a distance, of course, over the years, and I'm very proud of you.'

She smiled. 'I have you and father to thank for it. Without your encouragement . . .'

'Nonsense.' He wouldn't have it that he had contributed in any way to her achievements and she didn't embarrass him by pressing the issue. He proffered a plate of biscuits. 'If I had to have someone here as a locum I couldn't have chosen anyone I would have liked better. I was delighted when your father told me you'd qualified. It seemed absolutely opportune.'

She looked at him keenly. 'I gather your heart attack was quite severe and that you're likely to be convalescing for some time.'

He pulled a wry face. 'Well, so the doc days, but then, I never take any notice of what doctors say. I've heard it all before. I'm as strong as an ox, always was, and I don't intend to let them start telling me any different.'

She joined in with his laughter but wasn't fooled. The change in Tom Jameson had shocked her although she was careful not to let it show as she looked at the once stout frame, now much thinner, and saw the tell-tale bluish colouring around his mouth. Her throat tightened.

'How long is it before you're allowed to get back to work?'

His hand rose. 'They talk about three months. I

think they're playing safe and I've told 'em so. Nothing is going to keep me from my desk once I feel I can cope. But in the meantime I knew it wasn't fair to Grant to ask him to cope alone. He would have done, mind, Grant's a first class doctor I'm lucky to have him, especially as he could have specialised or gone to a much bigger practice than this.'

'Why didn't he?'

'I don't really know. He didn't volunteer any reasons and I didn't ask, probably if I'm honest because I was too glad to get him.' He sighed. 'But the fact is, I couldn't ask him to go on indefinitely taking normal surgeries as well as emergency calls and night visits, which is why I wrote to your father.'

Lee stared into her cup. 'I'm flattered that you should have thought of me, Uncle Tom, but you do realise I'm just fresh out of medical school with no experience behind me as yet?'

'My dear girl, how do you gain experience except by doing the job you were trained for? You have to start somewhere. Why not here?'

She laughed, exasperatedly. 'You're as bad as Father. The question is, how will your partner, Dr Sinclair, feel about it?'

'Grant trusts my judgment. In any case he got your letter and the mere fact that you trained at St Clements was enough to convince him.'

It didn't entirely dispel her doubts but she managed to hide them. 'I'm looking forward to meeting him.' She glanced at the small brass clock on the shelf just as the phone rang and Tom Jameson went to answer it.

'That's probably Grant now, on his way back to the surgery. I'll take you around and show you the set-up. Just let me tell him you've arrived.'

She helped herself to more tea as he spoke quickly and quietly to the voice she could hear at the other end of the phone. Her own name was mentioned. It was a brief conversation and Tom Jameson's face held a worried expression as he returned to the room.

'Trouble?'

'Mm, I'm afraid so. Some kind of emergency has cropped up and Grant is going to be delayed. It's a damned nuisance. Evening surgery starts in about an hour.'

Lee was already on her feet. 'Can I help? Just tell me what you want me to do.'

He looked at her, uncertainly. 'You've hardly had time to take your coat off.'

'Perhaps it's just as well,' she joked, reassuringly. 'Anyway, this is precisely what I came here for and as both you and Father have pointed out, it's best sometimes to leap straight in at the deep end.'

His look of doubt was tinged with undisguised relief. 'Well, if you're sure. Grant asked if you'd have any objection to starting the surgery. He'll get back as soon as possible.'

She did swift battle with a feeling of panic and said, brightly, 'No, of course I don't mind.' She was already reaching for her bag and gloves, feeling her heart thudding uncomfortably fast. 'Someone will have to show me where everything is.'

'I'll do that myself.' He was shrugging himself into his coat as she hesitated.

'Should you?'

He wound a scarf round his neck. 'Why not? I've no intention of allowing myself to become a permanent invalid. Besides, a little exercise is good for me. The surgery is about half a mile from here,' he explained as she drove the Mini, following his instructions. 'Grant lives in my house. It's a suitable arrangement. I have a housekeeper who cooks for both of us and who doesn't object to the erratic hours we keep. Here,' he leaned forward.

She turned the car into the drive-way and was quite pleasantly surprised to find a modern, single-storied building which proved as they entered to be light and airy as well as well-equipped. The waiting room was large, its walls painted in a nice pastel shade and she was pleased to see that there were some large green plants as well as bright chairs and several tables with magazines scattered over them.

Tom Jameson correctly interpreted her expression. 'It was built three years ago, just before Grant joined me.' He opened various doors. 'You'll see that we've gone in for a certain amount of patient comfort. I've heard doctors say they don't believe in encouraging patients to be ill. I feel that those who need to come should be able to sit in reasonable comfort and then be dealt with as efficiently as possible. You'll find the files there.' He indicated the reception area. 'Our receptionist Mrs Allen will be here any time now and so will the first patient.' He opened another door. 'This will be your surgery.'

She looked in at the room with its blue-carpeted floor and curtains which could be drawn round the examination couch. Crossing to the desk she put her bag down.

'Well, I suppose I'd better make a start. I just hope I don't let you down, Uncle Tom.'

'I'm sure there's no danger of that. Don't even think about it. You'll find our people quite a nice, human lot. Mind you,' his eyes twinkled, 'I'd like to see a few of their faces when they walk in and see you sitting behind that desk. Come to think of it, I reckon Grant may be in for a bit of a surprise too.'

He was gone before she had a chance to ask him why Grant Sinclair should be surprised and then she forgot about it completely as the first patient walked in. For the next hour she worked her way steadily through the list and was congratulating herself upon having survived comparatively unscathed when the door opened again.

Having been told that the last patient had gone she assumed, without looking up, that it was simply a late arrival. Completing the notes she was making, she smiled.

'Hullo, please sit down. I'll be with you in a moment.'

She heard the soft hiss of indrawn breath, then an

angry voice said, 'Just what's going on? Who the devil are you and what, may I ask, do you think you're doing in that chair?'

There was something about the autocratic tone which for one moment set her heart thudding sickeningly, then she found herself looking up into the darkly sombre eyes which regarded her with such open hostility. It wasn't possible. But as her gaze rose, agonisingly, from the roll neck sweater and tweed jacket to the taut face above it, premonition became reality and her face whitened.

'*You!*' The word broke from his lips as if he had uttered an oath.

She heard herself repeating his own word, praying even now that it might all prove to be some terrible mistake as she rose slowly to her feet and faced him. But it was no mistake. This was the man who had so rudely pushed her aside, who had dared to accuse her of practising amateurish first aid.

He faced her, his eyes narrowed. 'I'm waiting for an explanation.'

She swallowed hard. 'I'm here as locum to Dr Sinclair until Dr Jameson is recovered from his heart attack.' She resented the look of disbelief on his face.

'You can't be. I'm Dr Sinclair and I assure you I was expecting a Dr Forrester.'

'That's right. *I'm* Dr Forrester.'

His mouth was a grim line as he moved closer. 'But I was expecting a man.'

She felt a stab of resentment. 'Well, I'm sorry,

Doctor. I don't know why you should have gained that impression. Certainly I made no secret . . .' Her gaze wavered. 'Surely Tom must have told you?'

His mouth tightened. 'He talked to me, vaguely, about getting someone in. I didn't listen. I told him I could cope.'

'Well obviously he didn't think so, and perhaps you should have listened.'

'You signed your letter Dr Lee Forrester.'

Her chin rose. 'Naturally, because that happens to be my name. Surely there's no law against that? I imagine if you'd shown any interest Uncle Tom would have told you. It's hardly my fault if you weren't sufficiently concerned to ask.'

She found herself beginning to hate his arrogance and, even worse, to realise that she would never be able to work for a man like Grant Sinclair. It had all been a terrible mistake and he was losing no time in making it perfectly clear that he fully shared her view.

CHAPTER TWO

THE silence which stretched so long and ominously between them was broken as he slammed the door to a close behind him and advanced into the room.

Lee had to fight a sudden desire to run, digging her feet instead more firmly into the thick carpet. There was something definitely intimidating about Grant Sinclair. His mere presence seemed to fill the room. As she studied him more closely she realised that he was even taller than she had first imagined. Thinner too. In the street there had been no time to see the faint lines of tiredness edging his mouth, but they were there, adding a kind of ruthlessness which left her feeling vaguely shaky. Her gaze shifted quickly to his eyes. They were shadowed, evidence of the work load he had been carrying since Uncle Tom's heart attack, and, having dealt with only one surgery, she could understand why. Which made his opposition to her all the more unreasonable, she told herself, drawing in a steadying breath.

He ruffled a hand through his hair. 'There's obviously been some mistake. I don't know how this happened. Perhaps the position wasn't made clear.' He threw his jacket onto the chair where she had been sitting, and she stiffened at the proprietorial gesture.

'I'm afraid I don't see that there has been a mistake, Dr Sinclair, at least not as far as I'm concerned. There was no suggestion that you required a male partner, but in any case, surely you aren't objecting solely on the grounds of my sex. If so I find your attitude totally unreasonable and . . . incomprehensible.' She was aware of the two high spots of colour in her cheeks and his own angry expression.

'Oh, my God, not women's lib. Spare me that.'

The element of scorn in his tone rankled. 'If you'll forgive me for saying so, Doctor, *I* didn't raise the question of sex, you did, and totally without justification. May I remind you that I am a fully qualified doctor.'

'Newly qualified.'

Her lips tightened. 'But qualified, nonetheless.' She stood her ground, determined not to be browbeaten by his bullying tactics. 'I made it perfectly clear in my letter and I assumed that you must have spoken to Unc . . . Dr Jameson before offering me the job.'

'Naturally.' He was staring at her with the kind of cool speculation which made her feel oddly vulnerable. 'However, it seems he forgot to mention that you were a woman.'

'Possibly because he didn't consider it important,' she snapped, then bit her lip. 'The fact remains, I'm here and I came to do a job of work. Or are you trying to tell me that I'm not suitable?' For some reason her hand shook as she put the case notes she had been holding onto the desk.

His mouth compressed. 'That's precisely what I'm saying, and if I'd been made fully aware of the facts I would have made my feelings quite clear.'

Shock drew a stifled gasp from her. 'But that . . . that is unfair.'

'It's not unfair . . . Doctor. It's a statement of fact, however unpalatable.' His gaze raked over her. 'Just how old are you, Dr Forrester?'

'I'm twenty-five.'

Surprise flickered briefly over his features. 'You look about eighteen.'

'Well, I can hardly help that.'

'I don't suppose you can, but it's not likely to instil confidence in the patients, is it, when they walk in here and see you sitting behind that desk.'

The words were so close to those Uncle Tom had used that she flinched. 'My looks don't affect my abilities as a doctor.' She stabbed a finger at the pile of cards on the desk. 'I coped with a full list of patients and not one complained.' It wasn't exactly the truth. By the end of the list she had resigned herself to the wary looks which greeted her as each new patient walked in, and the almost inevitable words, 'But I'm Dr Sinclair's patient.' A little explanation seemed to have satisfied most doubts but Grant Sinclair's gaze barely passed over the cards.

'Oh sure. Go to the top of the class. Now you

know what being a GP is all about.' He frowned, then bent to shuffle through the pile. 'I was supposed to see Mrs Latimer tonight.'

'Yes, that's right.' She remembered the woman. 'She came in.'

He looked from her to the card, scanning the brief details she had written, then his eyes narrowed. 'You've reduced the dosage of her drugs?'

'That's right. I judged it to be appropriate.' Her voice was surprisingly calm.

'On what grounds?'

For a moment doubts surged only to be replaced by confidence in her own judgment. She had talked to the woman, discussed with her at length the new treatment which had been prescribed two weeks earlier and was satisfied, with reservations, that it was sound.

'She had obviously made progress but was complaining of side effects. I went over them carefully and everything pointed to the fact that the dosage was too high.'

He grunted. 'That's possible, I suppose. It was something I was watching pretty carefully particularly as that drug is still new.'

'Yes, I realised that. But since she had made progress a reduction in the dosage seemed appropriate rather than a change of drug.'

He looked at her. 'I agree, but I shall want to see her regularly for a while to be sure.'

'Naturally, I assumed you would. I asked her to be sure to make an appointment for next week and told her that in the meantime if she feels she needs to see someone before that, she should come to the surgery.'

He tossed the card back onto the desk and ruffled a hand through his hair. 'Well, I can't fault your actions, but that doesn't alter the facts. One evening surgery isn't general practice. You've seen the kind of area we have here. It's growing. We have the village as well as a developing community around it. It's growing fast. You must have seen the building that's going on. In a few more years we shall have lost our identity completely and been swallowed up by the town.' He crossed to the window, staring out into the darkness which had somehow crept up unnoticed as she had worked. 'It's like some wretched disease, it creeps insidiously and before you know it everything is changed.'

The note of bitterness in his voice shook her, yet she knew what he meant. Foxley was a beautiful village, but for how long?

'They call it progress.'

'Do they?' He whipped round, his mouth compressed into a narrow line. 'Well you and I have to bear the brunt of that progress, Dr Forrester, and I'm not at all sure that you're up to it. It means crowded surgeries, and being called out of your bed at night, sometimes for nothing more than a toothache.'

'That's what I trained for. I chose to do this work,' she added, defensively.

'So did Tom Jameson. Medicine is his life and look what it's done to him.'

She released her breath, wishing he hadn't reminded her. 'I know, but aren't you forgetting that he's also sixty-five and that he has always worked too hard because that's the kind of man he is?' She looked up into his face and felt a slight tremor run through her, triggered by an emotion she didn't choose to analyse. There was something about Grant Sinclair which made her feel that women were still chattels, that their proper place was in the home, caring for and catering to the needs of a man. It was a positively medieval notion and one she intended to shatter, which didn't quite explain why a mental vision of herself waiting for a man like Grant Sinclair to come home at night should flicker briefly into her mind. She pushed it away. 'I'm not here to try and take his place. I'm not crazy enough to imagine I could ever hope to fill his shoes. That's your job.' Her tone added, *'If you're capable of it.'* 'Mine is to help out for a few weeks and I think you at least owe it to me to let me try now that I'm here. It was hardly my fault that you mistook me for a man.'

His mouth twisted and the blood rushed hotly into her face as for several seconds his gaze slid over her slender figure, taking in the neat, woollen dress she was wearing. It was one of her favourites, or had been until now. Its delicate jade-green colouring suited her, but suddenly she was aware that it moulded to her figure in a way which a man like

Grant Sinclair might consider deliberately provocative.

'I'm sure I'm in no danger of making that mistake again.'

Her fingers fumbled clumsily at the buttons of the white coat, drawing them together, but his expression had already changed and his tone was sharp.

'I don't have much choice now that you're here, do I? Tom is right, though it took me a while to admit it, even to myself. If I'm going to do my job properly I do need help, as much to put his mind at rest as anything else. You've seen him. He's conscientious, if he thinks I can't give the patients two hundred per cent in his absence, he'll be back at his desk and dead within the month. I've tried, but I'm only human.'

She felt a surprising stab of pity. A man like Grant Sinclair wouldn't admit defeat easily.

'Well, at least I can relieve the pressure of some of the surgeries as well as taking my fair share of the night calls and visits.'

His glance was scornful. 'Believe me, Dr Forrester, if you take it on there won't be any half measures, but I give you a week, maybe two at most, and don't say I didn't warn you when you have to admit defeat. If you had any idea that this was going to be a cushy little number just because we're a village and you had good old Uncle Tom to pull a few strings you'd better forget it. This practice will either make or break you.'

She clenched her fists together, well aware of the mockery in his eyes and yet at the same time a feeling of relief swept over her. She was staying and despite Grant Sinclair she would prove that she was up to the job. Somehow she was determined to dispel Grant Sinclair's medieval arrogance towards women. Or was it just towards herself? She pushed the thought away. After all, his opinion of her wasn't important. If he could survive the next three months of working together then so would she. But suddenly there seemed very little pleasure in the prospect.

CHAPTER THREE

THE sound of someone tapping at the bedroom door brought Lee out of a heavy sleep. Instinctively she sat up, her hand reaching for a phone which wasn't there, then the door opened and the sight of her uncle's housekeeper, Mrs Dawson, carrying a tray of tea brought memory flooding back and with it a slight pang of alarm. She reached for her watch. 'Eight o'clock. Oh no!'

Mrs Dawson put down the tray, smiling. 'Now don't you worry, my dear.'

'But I should have been up hours ago.' Lee was feverishly pushing the covers back. 'At this rate I'm going to miss morning surgery, and on my first day too. Has Dr Sinclair left yet?'

'Oh bless you, yes, ages ago. He had a call, a child with suspected appendicitis, and he said it would hardly be worth coming back here by the time he'd finished so he was going straight to the surgery.'

'Damn.' Lee struggled grimly out of the mound of covers and wished crossly that she had unpacked properly the night before.

'I'm sure you needn't worry. He won't expect you to be there on your first morning.'

'I wouldn't count on it,' Lee muttered grimly

under her breath as she reached for a dressing gown and hastily drank the hot tea. 'He's probably gloating that I managed to oversleep.' Mercifully the tea brought her fully awake though she was still tired after the previous day's travelling, but that was something she was going to have to get used to and the sooner the better.

From the bottom of her half unpacked suitcase she brought out the sturdy alarm clock, wound it and set it. From now on she wasn't taking any chances.

'Breakfast will be ready as soon as you come down,' Mrs Dawson called from the doorway. 'Bacon and eggs and some nice toast and marmalade.'

'I'm afraid I won't have time.' Lee stuck her head round the bathroom door but the housekeeper was already disappearing down the stairs leaving Lee to take a hasty shower before dressing in a dress of soft, blue wool which set off her figure and colouring to perfection yet still looked formal enough for a day's work.

Hurrying downstairs she saw to her dismay that breakfast was indeed ready, and, to her chagrin, was even more dismayed to feel her stomach rumble noisily as the plate was put in front of her. Tom Jameson nodded approvingly over the morning newspaper. 'It pays to eat a good breakfast. Glad you're being sensible.'

'I'll just have to make sure I have more time to enjoy it in future.' She spooned sugar into her coffee. 'I didn't expect to see you down so early, Uncle Tom.'

'Can't abide lying in bed. Never done it, can't start now.' He passed the salt. 'It's funny how you get out of the habit. It's hard when you first start taking night calls. There were times when I would have given my right arm for a proper night's sleep, but you get used to it.'

Lee grimaced. 'Somehow I doubt if I'm going to get the chance. Dr Sinclair isn't going to be pleased when I fail to turn up on my first day. It was stupid of me, but I just assumed I would be called. Shades of being spoilt at home.' She cast a wary eye at the clock as she buttered a piece of toast. 'I may still just about make it.'

'There's no need. Grant's perfectly used to coping with morning surgery.'

'Yes, I'm sure he is, but he was called out in the early hours. A child with appendicitis, I think.'

'Mm, I thought I heard the phone, still, today won't be a long surgery, Tuesdays never are.'

'Oh?' She looked at him curiously. 'Why, what's special about Tuesdays?'

He grinned. 'The bus.'

'The bus?'

He laughed at her bewilderment. 'Market day in town. The bus runs specially. People in Foxley don't get ill on Tuesdays unless they can help it.'

'Oh, I see.' She laughed. 'Still, I'm here to do a job.'

'And I'm not disputing it, my dear. Grant works

hard and expects everyone else to do the same but he's fair and you did sit in for him last night at a moment's notice.'

'Yes, but that was the least I could do.' She gulped down the rest of her coffee and began hunting in her bag for her car keys, telling herself that she hadn't noticed any evidence of Grant Sinclair's fairness. 'Besides, I'll feel happier if I put in an appearance, Uncle Tom. I don't want any favours.' It would be just what Grant Sinclair was expecting, she thought, and she jolly well wasn't going to give him the chance to be proved right. 'I'd better dash.' Planting a kiss on Tom's cheek she rushed out to the Mini and headed down the road telling herself that the fluttering in her stomach was indigestion and not nerves.

In the event Margaret Allen the receptionist viewed her arrival with obvious surprise and relief. 'Oh, Dr Forrester, how nice! I didn't think you'd be in on your first morning. Dr Sinclair didn't mention it but I'm certainly glad you've turned up.'

No he wouldn't have mentioned it, Lee thought, but she smiled as she unbuttoned her coat. 'Actually, I have a confession to make. I overslept, but I have every intention of starting at the proper time in future. It's what I'm here for and I'd like to get into a proper routine as soon as possible.'

'Well, I can't say I'm sorry.' Margaret Allen ruefully indicated the pile of patients' case notes. 'We seem to have developed an epidemic.'

'What happened? I understood from Dr Jameson that Tuesdays were normally quiet.'

'Yes they are, but then he probably doesn't know that the bus has been cancelled because of the bad weather. The driver can't get through and even if he could there's a risk he may not be able to make the return journey.' She laughed. 'And apart from that I dare say the word has got round.'

'The word?'

Margaret Allen eyed her with amusement. 'In a place like this everyone knows what goes on, They'll have heard there's a new lady doctor and will want to come and look you over.'

Lee's eyes twinkled. 'That's a daunting prospect. Still, the sooner we satisfy their curiosity the better. Perhaps I'd better make a start.' Taking a handful of case notes she made her way into surgery and rang the bell for the first patient.

All in all the first morning passed remarkably quickly. There was a spate of sore throats, most of which could be treated with Disprin, though a few needed antibiotics to clear an infection. It was rewarding to be able to confirm the pregnancy of a young woman who had been trying for three years to have a baby. Watching her leave, Lee felt a tiny stab of emotion she had never experienced before, almost a feeling of . . . well it couldn't be jealousy, she told herself brusquely, her hand coming down sharply on the bell again.

The door opened slowly and, looking up from the notes she had just completed, Lee watched with amusement as an elderly figure muffled in thick coat, scarf and cap, edged his way round the door, regarding her suspiciously.

'Please do come in, Mr Watkins.' A quick glance at the card showed that the patient had a history of chronic bronchitis. She indicated the chair with a smile. Eddie Watkins however remained firmly at the door from where he grunted unhappily.

'I come to see Dr Sinclair. Don't want to see no female lady doctor. 'T'ain't proper.'

Lee hid a smile. 'Perhaps I can help?'

'I been under Dr Sinclair. I wants to see 'im about me bronichals, 'e knows all about 'em, 'e does.' He coughed wheezily and Lee felt her heart sink. This was the first patient who had actually refused to consult her and it was disconcerting. The wary glances she had expected but this was something else, and suppose they all started insisting on seeing Grant?

She smiled what she hoped was a reassuring smile. 'I know Dr Sinclair is a little busy this morning. That's why I'm here, to help out, just until Dr Jameson is well enough to take over again.'

Eddie Watkins grunted unhappily but ventured further into the room. Seen closer to she judged his age to be about seventy. 'Don't like choppin' and changin',' he complained. ''T'ain't right.'

'No, you're right, it is upsetting, but hopefully Dr Jameson should be well enough to come back in a few weeks' time. It's just that until then Dr Sinclair is finding the work load a little heavy and I'd like to be able to help.'

He sucked at his teeth and wheezed, noisily. 'I don't 'old with lady doctors. Told Tom Jameson so but he wouldn't 'ave it. Says you got to move with the times. I told him, I 'ad my time near enough and what weren't proper when I were young ain't proper now. Women got their place and it ain't messing about with men's bodies.'

Lee felt her lips quiver. 'I don't think my uncle would agree with you, Mr Watkins, especially not as it was he who first suggested I should take up medicine.'

Bushy eyebrows rose. 'Uncle? Tom Jameson your uncle?'

'Well, more or less,' she admitted, carefully, seeing the spark of interest. 'He's actually a good friend of my father's and I've known him all my life.'

Eddie Watkins eased himself into the chair and sighed a rattling sigh. He leaned forward and tapped the card on the desk in front of her. 'Well he knows me bronichals same as Dr Sinclair. I'll 'ave a bottle of the usual and some of them tablets.'

Lee studied the notes, trying to hide her confusion. The medication last prescribed was one she recognised as having been proved to be most beneficial in cases like Eddie Watkins where it was a matter of offering relief rather than a cure. She looked at the nicotine stained fingers and said nothing. At Eddie Watkins' age there was little chance of persuading him to change the habits of a lifetime. Instead, having questioned him gently, she wrote out a prescription. 'There we are, Mr Watkins, but I'd like you to come back in a week's time. You can make an appointment to see Dr Sinclair at the desk as you go out,' she said, hastily. He got to his feet, thrust the paper carelessly into a pocket and trundled out. She could hear him coughing as he made his way out into the street.

When the last patient had left she made her way to the receptionist's room to find Margaret Allen making coffee. There was no sign of Grant.

'You finished nice and early after all, Doctor. Heaven knows what it would have been like if you hadn't come along. Here we are,' she proffered a cup. 'Help yourself to sugar.'

Lee did so and said, wryly, 'I'm not sure every one of the patients I saw today would agree with you. Old Mr Watkins made it perfectly clear that he holds no truck with women doctors.'

'Oh Eddie, don't take any notice. Eddie Watkins likes a good moan, he thrives on it and women usually bear the brunt of it. He's all right really.'

'Actually I rather liked him, once I'd managed to fight my way past the initial barrier, but then, I expect it to take time. Medicine is such a personal business. People get used to their doctor. They don't like change. Not that I'm going to be here long enough for them to get used to me.' She drank her coffee, wondering why the thought should give her a sense of disappointment. She pulled herself up sharply. 'Now don't start getting attached to things,' she told herself, then the door opened and the likelihood vanished as Grant Sinclair's frowning glance raked her as she sat in the chair.

For some reason she found herself fighting a feeling of guilt, which was quite ridiculous because she had done a good morning's work and earned a coffee break. Purposely she relaxed, ignoring him as she bent her head over the *Medical Journal*.

'Is that the lot?' He sounded cross and ruffled a hand through the thatch of dark brown hair.

Margaret Allen nodded with a twitch of humour in her eyes as she glanced in Lee's direction. 'It wasn't as bad as I expected. It's a good job Dr Forrester came in. Here we are, Doctor, your coffee.' She handed him a cup. He took it, glancing at his watch.

'I don't know that I really have time. How many visits are there?'

'Six, Doctor.'

He took the list, scanning it as he drank his coffee. 'Mm, three look pretty routine. This one, Mr Collins, I'd better do first. I've not been too happy about him for some time. His arthritis is getting to the point where we're going to have to get him into hospital to get that hip joint done.'

'If you can persuade him, that is.' Margaret's smile was resigned.

'Well I'll just have to give it another try.' He put his empty cup down. Margaret gathered them up and took them away and Lee found herself waiting, irritably, for some sign that he had even noticed her presence. Eventually, when it seemed it wasn't forthcoming, she rose to her feet.

'I'm sorry I was late in,' she said, carefully. 'You should have called me.'

His gaze was directed, frowning, from the list to her face. 'It didn't occur to me that you'd need it, but don't let it worry you. I didn't expect you in this morning anyway.'

She felt her temper rise. 'Why not? I thought I'd made it perfectly clear last night that I was here to do a job.'

'Don't let it worry you. I'll see to it that you do, Doctor.'

The note of contempt in his voice made her flinch. 'Then suppose we start straight away.'

'Fine.'

She bit her lip. 'Look, I'm perfectly capable of taking my share of the calls.'

He raised an eyebrow. 'You really think you know the area well enough?'

'I can read a map.'

'Really? Then you must be one of the few women who can.'

She drew in a breath but refused to let herself be drawn. 'As it happens I've already had a look at a detailed map of the immediate area. Once I know the addresses I can look them up. In any case I do have a tongue in my head.'

'Now that I don't doubt.'

She wasn't sure whether it was sarcasm or laughter that filled his eyes but she felt the colour scorch her cheeks. 'I'm perfectly serious. I could take half those calls.'

'And I'm being serious too, Dr Forrester. One reason I didn't make a point of insisting you come in to take surgery this morning was because I imagined you'd make use of the time to get to know your way around, and also because normally on Tuesdays we only have one doctor on duty anyway, even when Tom was fit.'

Lee swallowed hard, feeling suddenly rather foolish. 'I see. Well I'm sorry I didn't realise that, but in any case today was obviously an exception.'

'I'm not saying I'm not grateful.'

'I'm not asking for your gratitude, Dr Sinclair,' she snapped, crossly. 'I just ask to be allowed to do my share. Just forget I'm a woman.'

His mouth twisted, sardonically. 'That might be rather difficult.'

'I'm trying to be serious, Doctor.' Her eyes glittered angrily and she realised that he was laughing at her.

'I'm sure you are.'

'Then please get it into your head that I am not only willing, but perfectly capable of doing my job and doing it well. I know you didn't want me here, but now that I am it will be better for both of us if we accept the situation and make the best of it. After all, it's only likely to be for a few weeks anyway. I think I can stick it if you can.'

He stood looking at her and she was suddenly uncomfortably aware of him as a man, an attractive man. Not that she liked the type herself, of course. Grant Sinclair was too overbearing. Still, she could see that some women might be impressed by the tall, lean good looks.

His mouth tightened. 'As far as Tom's concerned it will only be a few weeks.'

Her eyes widened. 'I don't understand. Surely you're not saying . . .'

'I'm saying that Tom believes what he wants to believe. He's made up his mind he's going to get back to work.'

'And are you saying he won't?' She felt a cold stab of fear as he looked at her almost pityingly.

'I'm saying that he's more ill than he realises or chooses to realise.'

For a minute she was bereft of speech. 'But I thought he was getting over the heart attack. He seemed so well when I spoke to him.'

'I'm sure he did. But then, he knew you were coming. I'd suggest you reserve your judgment until you've seen him when he's tired or you catch him off guard.'

She stared at him, bleakly, not wanting to believe. Her mouth felt dry. 'Just how bad is he?' And then, as he didn't answer, 'Look, I have a right to know. He and my father have been friends for a very long time. He's always been like a real uncle to me.'

He frowned. 'It's not good. The attack was worse than he realises and he could have another at any time.'

'And he doesn't know?' She looked at him askance.

'If he does he's not letting on.' His mouth tightened, grimly. 'Can't you understand, Tom's work is his life. If he has to give that up he may as well be dead as far as he's concerned. For heaven's sake, why do you imagine when he started talking even vaguely about taking on an assistant that I tried to talk him out of it?'

She stared at him uneasily. 'But how long do you think you could have gone on carrying the workload alone?'

'I would have managed somehow. In the end I gave in because Tom had convinced himself in his own mind that it really wouldn't be for more than a few weeks.'

She swallowed hard. 'And now you're saying that isn't true?'

'You want me to be honest or wrap it up nicely for you?'

She flinched and felt the tears well up, stinging at her eyes. How could he be so cold blooded, so cruel? 'Just what exactly is the prognosis?'

'You're a doctor, you must have a pretty good idea.'

He was right. She just didn't want to have to put it into words. But how could she insist in one breath that she was capable of doing her job if she was going to burst into tears and go all feminine on him at the first hurdle. She straightened her shoulders and faced him. 'And what if he doesn't go back to work, takes things easily?'

His face was grim as he bent to pick up the case notes Margaret had left on the table. 'Then he could go on for years, but Tom isn't the sort to take things easy, you must know that.'

'So what do we do?'

'The only thing we can do. Carry on. One way or another Tom is eventually going to come to terms with it.'

'But wouldn't it be kinder to tell him the truth?'

'Do you want to be the one to do it? Tell him he should start living the life of an invalid?'

She flinched. 'No . . . I suppose I don't.'

His mouth twisted. 'No, it's not that easy is it, Doctor.' He eyed her scornfully, but she wasn't going to be put off.

'I don't see that anything is solved by our arguing or by your constant resentment of me. I'm here . . .'

'And I'd better learn to put up with you, hadn't I, Doctor?'

Lee drew herself up, shaking with anger. 'You aren't the only person who has feelings. I happen to care for Tom too, very much as it happens, and I intend doing what I can to help whether you like it or not. But just what do I have to do to prove to you that I'm capable?'

'Don't bother. I'm not asking you to prove anything.'

'Aren't you?' Her voice shook. 'Then perhaps it's just me, as a woman, that you resent. Well I'm afraid there's not a lot I can do about that, but you needn't worry, I'll pull my weight, starting with taking half those calls.' She held out her hand. 'You take three, I'll take three.'

There was a momentary pause, then he flicked three cards out of the pile, tossing them onto the table in front of her. 'If there's one thing I can't abide, it's a domineering woman. One of these days someone is going to teach you a lesson, Dr Forrester, and it might come as something of a shock.'

She gasped. 'And if there's one thing I can't stand, it's arrogant, over-bearing, woman-hating . . .' She stifled the rest as the door opened and Margaret Allen beamed round the door.

'Oh, Dr Sinclair, there was a telephone call for you. I knew you were probably in conference with Dr Forrester so I took a message. Miss Latimer called and said she would be delighted to meet you for dinner this evening.'

Lee felt the colour in her cheeks deepen. She was briefly aware of the mocking stare as she scooped up the case notes and marched quickly out of the room. It was galling to find herself wondering just who the mysterious Miss Latimer was. Probably seventy, large and tweedy. 'Just his type' she told herself, but somehow the image she had conjured up didn't seem to fit and the knowledge rankled.

She pushed the thoughts firmly aside as she climbed into the car. After all she wasn't in the least bit interested in Grant Sinclair or his love life. She was here to do a job and she would do it in spite of him. The gears grated and she swore under her breath, all too aware of the tall figure standing at the window, no doubt laughing his male chauvinist head off.

CHAPTER FOUR

WHETHER by accident or design, and from the little she already knew of Grant Sinclair it was probably the latter, she found herself covering miles in order to get to the three calls, and even when she had eventually found them, the first two turned out to be fairly minor cases.

Consulting the list she made for the third which proved to be at the far end of a long, narrow lane. 'I'll bet he's done this on purpose,' she thought, grimly manoeuvring the car between low hedgerows until it finally brought her to Greystone Farm.

The patient turned out to be a fractious child who was obviously running a temperature.

'I'm so sorry to call you out, Doctor,' the anxious young woman kept insisting as she ushered Lee into the large, cosy front room where a huge fire blazed. 'Only it's so difficult to get to the surgery in my condition when John's got the car, and young Tracy here seems to have quite a high temperature.'

Lee smiled. 'Don't worry about it, Mrs Cox.' She put her bag down beside the chair before she moved to the comfortable old couch where the child lay. It didn't need an examination to tell her that it was a text-book case of german measles, but she made the usual investigations examining the bright, pin-prick spots and feeling for the raised glands. It was reassuringly straightforward.

'Well, at least you'll be pleased to know it isn't serious, just a dose of german measles. There's a lot of it around right now.'

The woman's tired face relaxed into a smile. 'Oh yes, I know, half the class at the local school have got it, only I wasn't sure and there's nothing worse than hauling a screaming, spotty child to the surgery.'

Lee turned her attention briefly from the child as Anne Cox sank into a chair and frowned, pressing a hand to her back.

'Well don't worry about it,' Lee said. 'You did the right thing in this case. Tracy has obviously got quite a nasty dose, but you'll find she will start to pick up again quite quickly in the next twenty-four hours. The worst time always seems to be when the first spots appear.'

The woman smiled her relief, then her expression changed to one of curiosity as she eyed Lee's smart brown coat and a fur hat perched cossack style on her head. 'You're new here aren't you? I'd heard Dr Jameson hasn't been well.' Her smile became suddenly taut as she got to her feet and closed her eyes, easing her back with her hand.

Watching her, a sudden warning bell began to clang in Lee's head. Tucking a blanket round the now sleeping child she asked, calmly, 'When's the baby due, Mrs Cox? I expect you must be getting pretty excited.'

The woman's laughter was strained as she leaned on one hand against the chair and it was some seconds before she answered. 'Excited's not the word, Doctor. Bored and frustrated is more like it. The last few weeks are always the worst. I feel like a cow, shapeless . . . well, all the wrong shape, full of milk and a . . .' she bit her lip, 'a wretched back ache.'

Lee felt her heartbeats switch into second gear. Glancing at the clock she saw that it was past lunch time and beginning to snow quite heavily again. 'I suppose you'd think it very rude of me if I asked if I could possibly have a cup of tea?'

Anne Cox's expression immediately became one of concern. 'Oh heavens no, of course I wouldn't. In fact I would have offered only I wasn't sure if you'd have the time.'

Lee grinned. 'Well normally I wouldn't, but as you're my last call and I'm going to be late getting back to Foxley anyway . . . It's my own fault. I'm not used to the area and I've probably gone miles out of my way to find places.'

'Well you sit down and get warm and I'll make the tea now.'

Lee hesitated. 'I'll tell you what, you tell me where the kitchen is and I'll make the tea while you keep an eye on young Tracy here. It will only take me a minute.'

Relief flooded over the woman's face as she eased herself carefully down into the chair. 'If you're sure you don't mind.'

'Not at all.' Mentally Lee made a note of the time as she stacked cups, saucers, sugar and milk onto the tray and waited for the kettle to boil. She made the tea and carried it back to the sitting room just in time to see Anne Cox sitting upright in the chair, her eyes closed and her hands gripping the chair arms. Lee put down the tray, her suspicions confirmed as the woman opened her eyes again, smiled apologetically and exhaled deeply.

'It's the baby, isn't it?' Lee said.

She nodded, her grip relaxing gradually as the contraction passed. 'But it shouldn't be. Not for another three weeks. Perhaps it's a false alarm.'

'It could be, but I think I'd better check you over, just in case,' Lee said, with gentle briskness. 'Babies have an annoying habit of not always sticking to dates.'

'Oh yes, I know, my first was two weeks early, but at my last clinic appointment they said everything was fine.'

'I'm sure it is. Three weeks isn't anything to worry about. The baby looks a pretty good size and he's probably just eager to get on with it.' But from the expression in the woman's eyes as she made a swift examination this one was in something of a hurry.

As she washed her hands Anne Cox breathed her way through another contraction and Lee glanced at her watch again. 'Well, it's definitely started. I think the best thing we can do is organise some help. Where are you booked to have the baby?'

'At the maternity unit in town.' Her eyes widened. 'But I don't think I'm going to make it.' Her hands gripped the chair again.

'Have you a phone?'

'Over there.'

'Fine, I'm going to ring for an ambulance and then if you can tell me where to get in touch with your husband he can take over young Tracy for a while. In the meantime is there a neighbour just in case the ambulance arrives before your husband?'

'There's Carol, at the next farm.'

'Okay, just give me her number. I'll see to it while you toddle upstairs and get your things together.'

She moved to the phone, dialled the number of the local maternity unit and asked for an ambulance. Sister's voice was brisk but apologetic.

'We'll do our best, Doctor, but the drivers are having a hard time. The roads are terrible with this fresh snow falling on top of the ice. Just hang on, we'll try and get to you.'

Lee smiled ruefully at the receiver. 'I will, Sister, but I'm not sure I can say the same for Mrs Cox.' She hung up, rang the number of Mr Cox's accountant where he had an appointment and finally the neighbour. Within minutes Carol Blake was at the door and Lee was relieved to find her both helpful and efficient.

'I'm glad you could come,' Lee explained as they went into the sitting room. 'I've sent for an ambulance but I doubt if it's going to get here in time. If you can cope with Tracy when she wakes up?'

'Just leave her to me, Doctor. We get along fine. If necessary I'll take her over to my place and feed her with my brood until things get back to normal.'

Lee smiled her gratitude. She had rolled up her sleeves and was on her way back upstairs when Anne Cox's voice called, waveringly.

'D . . . doctor. Oh . . . oh.'

Lee's feet flew. She moved mechanically, praying everything was going to be straightforward and that the ambulance would arrive within the next few minutes.

In the event, the ambulance driver came up the stairs and knocked on the bedroom door just as Lee was wrapping a sturdy, red-faced infant in a blanket and placing it in its mother's arm.

Jack Morecroft grinned. 'Sorry we were late, Doctor, but it looks as if you did pretty well without us.'

'Mrs Cox did very well.' She looked at the weary but triumphant young woman in the bed and pronounced as a flushed young man rushed through the door, 'Congratulations, Mr Cox, you have a super, eight pound daughter and she and her mum are doing very nicely.' She picked up her bag and eyed the happy group. 'There's nothing more I can do here for now. Everything was perfectly straightforward. I'll contact your midwife and let her know what's happened and she'll be out to see you and the baby later today.'

'Doctor,' Anne Cox called her as she reached the

door. 'Thank you, for everything. I don't know what I'd have done if you hadn't been here.'

'I expect you'd have managed, but let's just say young Tracy's german measles was a piece of very good timing. Come to think of it, that little lady is going to have a rather nice shock when she finally wakes up and realises she has a brand new sister. Anyway,' she glanced at her watch, 'I'd better be off.'

She left them to it, a contented group, slightly bewildered but obviously happy. It wasn't until she was driving back along the lanes that she realised she was actually very tired. Giving birth was an exhausting business, she thought, for everyone concerned.

It had stopped snowing but the late afternoon sky was leaden as the temperature dropped rapidly and she guessed it was already freezing hard. She had telephoned the surgery earlier, just to let Margaret Allen know the developments at Greystone Farm and to check that there were no more calls. Luckily there hadn't been, just a message from Grant to remind her that there was no evening surgery but that she would be on call. The thought of an evening in by the fire was suddenly very appealing and she found herself hoping that she wouldn't be called out. She wondered vaguely what Grant Sinclair did on his evenings off and remembered with sudden and totally irrational depression that he was dining out with Miss Latimer. Well good luck to the poor girl.

Her hands tightened on the wheel as the car lurched unsteadily against the rutted ice. It was a minor road, overhung by trees so that the pale sun hadn't penetrated during the day and it was making driving a nightmare. She should have checked the map to see if there was a more direct route but it hadn't occurred to her and it was too late now.

She shivered. The car's heater had been behaving erratically for weeks and she had meant to get it seen to but there had never seemed to be time and now the windscreen was icing up, obscuring her vision of the road ahead. Uneasily she realised that it was probably going to be dark in less than an hour's time and thought longingly of a bowl of hot soup. The vision evaporated sharply as the car spun wildly out of control. She fought desperately with the wheel, heard a vicious jarring sound and felt a thud which threw her forward in the seat, leaving her breathless and shaking. For some seconds she sat with her head lowered, her hands braced against the wheel, wondering what on earth had happened. The engine was still throbbing gently but when she eased the accelerator nothing happened and with a sinking feeling she switched off and climbed out to investigate.

What she saw drew an involuntary gasp of dismay from her. 'Oh no, it can't be, not here.' Her gaze rested miserably on the tyre. It was flat and wedged against a fallen tree trunk, half in, half out of a ditch. In fact, she shuddered at the realisation, she had been lucky. A few inches more and the car would have tipped down into what was probably a drop of about two feet. As it was it seemed like little consolation. Somehow she was going to have to change the wheel or get help and on a lonely stretch of road like this, that possibility seemed highly unlikely.

Slamming the door to a close, the mere thought of Grant Sinclair made her cringe. He was going to love it, she thought, crossly flinging the boot open and hunting for the wrench and a jack. Well, she wasn't going to give him the chance. The tools landed with a dull thud in the layer of snow and she struggled breathlessly with the spare tyre, blowing on numbed fingers.

It was difficult manoeuvring the jack into place. The ground was uneven but with an effort she managed it. Her fingers struggled with the wrench. One of the nuts came loose fairly easily but the second stuck and no amount of effort would shift it. She sat in the snow, tears of angry frustration blinding her. 'Oh, come on now.' The sound of her own voice startled her and she sniffed, rubbing a gloved hand across her frozen nose. But it was no good. The garage mechanic who had last changed the wheel had done a good job and her own hands were too cold and not strong enough to shift the nuts even by a fraction.

Resignedly she got to her feet, feeling her mouth quiver. She was tired and cold and, if she admitted it, scared too. With darkness falling and no specific idea of where she was or how far it was from Foxley it would be utter stupidity to try walking in these conditions.

She leaned against the car, staring at the open snow-covered fields. Her breath fanned white into the air and she hugged her arms about herself to stop the violent shivering which was probably shock as much as the cold. Her head ached where it had been caught a glancing blow as the car swung round and she thought longingly of the cosy fireside awaiting her arrival at Uncle Tom's. 'If I ever get there,' she muttered. 'I could die of cold out here, and for all Grant Sinclair cares, he probably hasn't even noticed I'm not back yet and even if he has he's more than likely just furious, wondering how I can have taken so long to make three simple calls.

'Blast the man,' she snapped, irritably, fighting the uncomfortable knowledge that, at that precise moment, she would be more than happy to see him come striding towards her, arrogantly taking charge.

Shivering she got back into the car and sat, trying to think rationally. If she sat here all night she would probably freeze to death. It was only a small road, the locals probably avoided it and larger traffic would certainly never make it. Dragging the map from the glove compartment she spread it out on her knees and tried to get her bearings. She had come too far to try walking back to Greystone Farm and Foxley was not quite as far in the opposite direction.

'Which leaves only one choice.' She refolded the

map grimly. 'I start walking towards Foxley and even at a conservative estimate that means a hike of about five miles. Oh well, thank God for sensible footwear.'

She climbed out again, collected her bag and started walking. With a bit of luck there might be a house or a telephone. Confidence vanished however as she battled for the first mile and a glance at her watch showed it had taken nearly an hour. Struggling against the cold wind she kept her head lowered, gritted her teeth and forced herself to keep going. At this rate it was going to take half the night and with horror she remembered that she was on call.

Her clothes were wet and her hands and feet numb with cold when she first heard the sound of a car engine. It was behind her, or perhaps she had imagined it. She turned, shading her eyes against the fine, powdery snow which was falling again and felt her heart sink. Nothing, nothing at all. Drained emotionally and physically she turned back the way she had been walking, fighting down the lump in her throat. Then, suddenly, there were definitely headlights cutting through the darkness and she heard herself laugh with relief. So she hadn't imagined it. There was a car. Slipping in her eagerness, she sat heavily in the snow and felt too tired to get up. Her hands covered her face, trying to instil some warmth into her frozen features as, out of the leaden darkness, the headlights slid over her, brakes were jammed on and a door slammed.

Dimly, as she stared through the curtain of snow, she saw a figure striding towards her, but only as a pair of hands dragged her bodily to her feet did she come fully awake to stare into a face that was taut with anger and which she recognised only too well, despite the wave of dizziness which was stealing rapidly over her. She noticed with a kind of irrationality that she could only put down to tiredness, that flakes of snow had settled in his hair and that he was wearing an old sweater. She trembled as he shook her.

'For God's sake, you little fool. Just what the hell do you think you're doing?'

Her teeth rattled. 'I was walking . . .'

'I can see that.' He was staring down at her, his eyes dark and angry, his fingers biting cruelly into her flesh. 'I found your car empty, about a mile back there.'

Her head jerked back with the force of his shaking and she shouted at him, suddenly angry. 'I must have hit some ice, it spun off the road and hit the ditch.' She gestured vaguely, suddenly too tired to argue. 'I couldn't change the wheel.' She gulped down a sob.

'You little idiot.' He was breathing hard. 'Have you any idea what . . .'

She dragged herself from his grasp. 'I told you it was an accident. You don't imagine I chose to get stranded out here, do you?'

'Frankly I wouldn't put anything past you. Why the devil didn't you phone for help?'

'From where?' she screamed in retaliation. 'And anyway I don't need your help. Will you let go of me.' She fought as his hands imprisoned her but this time he didn't release her. Instead his grip tightened.

'Don't be a little fool. You realise you might have been killed?'

'Well don't pretend you would have cared.' She knew she sounded hysterical but somehow she couldn't stop. His mouth was a grim line as he moved closer.

She was breathing hard. If only she didn't feel so weak, so dizzy.

'You're not making any sense, I suppose you realise that.' He pulled her closer his gaze searching. 'Are you sure you weren't hurt back there.'

'Of course I am. I'm perfectly all right.'

'You don't look it.'

Her eyes widened. 'Look, I don't need any favours from you, Doctor. If you hadn't come along I would have managed perfectly well.'

'Like hell you would.' She became conscious of the warm, masculine strength of him as he pulled her closer. She felt the cruel tightening of his fingers but he ignored her protesting whimper, his eyes glittering angrily. 'Just what is it that you're trying to prove, you little idiot?'

She gasped, refusing to acknowledge the crazy electric current which seemed to be running through her as her body was forced into contact with his. Her voice sounded unnatural as she tried to push him away. 'Prove? You're crazy. Why on earth should I need to prove anything, to you of all people.'

'I've no idea, suppose you tell me.' His head moved closer, his mouth barely a breath away from her own. She tried to turn away but his hand held her, forcing her closer and closer.

'Just because I'm a woman . . .' She broke off with a cry of pain.

'Well let's start by proving that.' Even as her lips parted in a gasp of pain his mouth came down on hers imprisoning it in a kiss which was both expert and brutal. He dragged her tightly to him. She tried to struggle but it was useless. The more she fought the more demanding the kiss became until her lips parted and she clung to him, sobbing a little as the barriers of resistance seemed to melt away. Her legs felt incredibly weak, his mouth was hard against her yielding lips and a slight moan of pleasure escaped her.

He released her abruptly, and with a finality which was as cruel as the kiss itself had been. She swayed. In spite of the freezing temperature she felt hot and brushed a hand against her forehead. With a muttered oath he caught her up in his arms and stared down at her.

'You're a stubborn creature, Dr Forrester.'

She wanted to say that she wasn't in the least stubborn but she felt too tired and far too comfortable in his arms, then he was striding back to the car and she felt herself being bundled into the passenger seat and a rug wrapped so tightly round her that she couldn't have moved even if she had wanted to.

'Where are we going? she asked as he climbed in beside her and started the engine. 'What about my car? We can't just leave it there.'

'We don't have any choice.' He didn't even spare a backward glance as his gaze concentrated grimly on the road ahead. 'Unless you imagine I'm going to try and haul it out of that ditch single-handed and in total darkness.' He turned to look at her. 'And even if I did, I assure you I wouldn't even consider allowing you to drive—not in the condition you're in. You're not safe to be let out alone, let alone behind the wheel of a car.'

Her fingers clawed at the confining rug. She wished she could slap his arrogant face. 'Then just where are we going?'

'Back to my place. It's not far from here and the sooner you get out of those wet things the better.'

He wasn't looking at her, which was just as well or he might have seen the tide of colour which washed up into her cheeks. 'Your place? Don't you mean Uncle Tom's?'

'I mean my place, Doctor. As it happens I have a small cottage about a mile from here. I don't use it very often but it's kept aired just in case I ever need it.'

She gritted her teeth. Just in case he ever wanted to take Miss Latimer there more likely. Well she wasn't Miss Latimer and had no intention of walking into his parlour. She stared at him through the darkness.

'There's no need for that. I'm perfectly all right. Just take me back to Uncle Tom's.'

'On the contrary, if you don't get out of those wet things quickly you're likely to end up with a dose of pneumonia.'

'Rubbish,' she snapped. 'All I need is a good long soak in a hot bath and some food, which I can get at Uncle Tom's.' Her heartbeat quickened as she saw his gaze shift from the road ahead to rake over her burning cheeks.

'You don't need to worry, Doctor, I'm quite convinced you're a woman. I don't have to carry you off to my lair and rape you to find out. Anyway, as it happens I have to go to the cottage to collect some papers.'

She drew back in the seat and realised as the car eventually came to a halt that her hands were actually clenched.

He helped her out but left the rug draped over her shoulders as he unlocked the cottage door. Inside she blinked as he switched on the lights and when her eyes had adjusted was surprised to discover that it was quite beautiful and attractively furnished. She stood shivering as he threw wood onto a fire which had obviously been lit earlier and within minutes a warm glow filled the room. Grant moved through to the kitchen, calling out, 'The bedroom's over there. Slip out of those things and help yourself to anything you need. There should be some old jeans and a shirt. I expect they'll be on the large side, but improvise. I'm sure you're good at it. You've got five minutes, then I'll bring the coffee in.'

Lee didn't move. Her feet felt glued to the floor. Only as he disappeared into the kitchen did she force herself to go into the bedroom and for some reason her heart thudded wildly as she saw the large bed. It looked comfortable and far too big for one man. She sat on it, huddled in the wet clothes, feeling suddenly overwhelmingly conscious of her own vulnerability. But why? It didn't make sense. She stared, trembling, around the room, hugging the blanket around her and was still there when Grant appeared in the doorway carrying two cups of coffee. His face darkened and he advanced, putting the cups down.

'I thought I told you to get out of those wet clothes.'

Her teeth chattered and she had to clamp them together. She wasn't even cold. It was ridiculous and so were the tears which suddenly oozed onto her cheeks.

In one swift movement his arms were round her. The contact sent a flame of desire rushing through her. It was ludicrous, just as she knew it was quite useless. He didn't even want her here, he had made that perfectly clear, and there was Miss Latimer.

'Lee.' His voice rasped hoarsely as his lips moved over her mouth.

She flinched, willing him to let her go before she

made a complete fool of herself. He did so abruptly, misinterpreting her response and said, icily, 'I thought I'd made it perfectly clear that you don't need to be afraid of me. I've no designs whatsoever upon your virtue, Dr Forrester.'

She couldn't speak. Her pulse was racing crazily and her head was spinning.

'You need some food.' His voice was curt. 'I'll go and fix some and this time you get out of those clothes, is that clear?' He stared at her and his expression darkened as she didn't move. 'For God's sake don't stand there like that or I may change my mind, then we'd both be sorry.'

The door slammed and after a moment she managed to pull herself together and began to struggle out of her clothes. When he returned she was wearing a bath robe she had found behind the door. It was several sizes too large and she had had to wind it round her waist. It made her look even slimmer and she was conscious of her hair clinging in damp tendrils to her head. But Grant Sinclair hardly seemed to notice. In fact he scarcely looked at her at all and when he spoke she couldn't miss the note of impatience in his voice.

'I've made an omelette. Help yourself and you'll find anything else you might need in the kitchen.'

She stared at him. 'But . . . aren't you going to eat too?'

'I don't have time. I have to get back to the surgery. I told you I only came here to collect some papers.'

She brushed aside a feeling of abject misery. 'But I'm supposed to be on call.'

'You're hardly in a fit state.' His look was scathing. 'I'll take care of it.'

'But your date . . . with Miss Latimer.'

'There'll be plenty of other times,' he said, shortly. 'I'll send a taxi out for you in a couple of hours.'

She didn't move. 'Thank you.'

'Don't thank me. Just eat.' He looked at her steadily then turned abruptly and a minute later she heard him drive away.

CHAPTER FIVE

LEE went down to breakfast the next morning with a tight feeling in the pit of her stomach. Having steeled herself to come face to face with Grant, it was something of an anti-climax then to find that he had already eaten and left. 'Probably as anxious to avoid me as I am him,' she told herself as she sat down and helped herself to tea and toast, keeping a wary eye on the clock.

Tom Jameson came in looking tired and even though he sounded cheerful enough Lee now found herself looking beyond the exterior appearance and not liking what she saw. Which made it all the more galling when she had to admit that Grant was right. No amount of persuasion, gentle or otherwise, was going to make the old man change the habits of a lifetime and Lee wasn't even sure that it would be wise to try. The life of an invalid would hold no charms for a man who had been as active as Tom.

He eyed her as she poured tea. 'I hear you had a spot of trouble yesterday.'

'Trouble?' her hand shook.

'Yes, pass the toast please. It was a marvellous piece of luck you being there. Mind you, we weren't anticipating any trouble. Annie Cox is as healthy as they come and her babies obviously arrive early as a matter of course.'

Lee felt a quick stab of relief as she realised her thoughts had been on a very different track altogether. 'Oh yes, it was a beautiful little girl and I hate to admit it but it gave me quite a thrill to deliver it.'

'Why hate to admit it? My dear girl, don't ever be afraid of sentiment. We may be doctors but we're still human and giving birth is still nature's finest miracle.'

Her eyes sparkled. 'You're right. I wouldn't have missed it for the world.'

Tom was busy rifling through a pile of mail which lay on the table. He handed a letter to her. 'This came for Grant after he'd left. Perhaps you'd take it in with you. I've a feeling he's waiting for it.'

'Yes, of course I will.' She put it in her bag. 'He must have left early this morning.'

'And not exactly in the best of moods either, according to Mrs Dawson, but I expect he'll get over it, whatever it is.'

The toast suddenly tasted like chaff in Lee's mouth. She washed it down hurriedly with tea and said, evenly, 'Uncle Tom, I've been thinking. I'm very comfortable here, you know that, but I've been toying with the idea of getting a flat. Nothing elaborate, and obviously it would have to be within easy reach of the practice, but . . . well it's just an idea.' She watched for his reaction and was relieved when he didn't take any apparent exception to the idea. On the contrary, he looked at her with a certain amusement.

'You're not asking for my approval are you, because if so, you know you don't need it. You're a grown woman, my dear, and whilst I feel a certain responsibility it certainly doesn't extend to trying to tell you how or where to live. You're old enough to make your own decisions.'

The words reminded her a shade too clearly of the previous evening and she winced. 'No, I'm not asking for your approval exactly, Uncle Tom, but I'd like to think you were quite happy about the idea. Of course I realise I'm only here on a temporary basis, but it would give me a bit more space and freedom to spread a little. You know how it is.' She smiled, hesitantly. It would also mean she didn't have to keep coming into contact with Grant. In fact, if she had a place of her own the only time they would need to meet would be at the practice and that should suit them both. The idea had come to her in the early hours of the morning after hours of tossing and turning and trying without much success to put the memory of that kiss out of her mind. Telling herself it had meant nothing didn't help. The only way she would be able to stay here and work was if she kept a safe distance between herself and Grant Sinclair and suddenly the idea of a flat had seemed the perfect solution. 'I just wanted to be sure you didn't feel that partners or assistants should live here for any particular reason,' she finished lamely.

'As a matter of fact I think a flat would be a good idea.' He ladled marmalade onto his toast and scattered crumbs as he gestured around the room. 'We're a bit cramped here and it does tend to be a bit of a bachelor establishment. Not that that's likely to be a permanent state in Grant's case, but for the moment he finds it convenient to live here.' He studied the remaining letters and frowned. 'He has the cottage, of course. Bought it when he first moved down here but never actually moved in for some reason. A bit lonely I dare say, and men don't tend to manage as well on their own as women, do they? Need someone to keep us in order.'

Lee lowered her head over the piece of toast she was buttering and muttered something.

'Anyway, if you're really serious, there's a chap I know has an agency in town. I'll let you have his address. He'll help you out if you give him some idea of what you want. Better still, I'll give him a call if you like and tell him you'll be dropping in, then he can have some details ready for you.'

'Would you really? That's marvellous. I could go this afternoon.'

'Shouldn't think you'd have any trouble finding something. If not a flat then a small cottage. People tend to come down here in the summer but at this time of year there are usually places to be had on a short lease.'

It sounded so perfect that she couldn't suppress a tiny tremor of excitement. With a bit of luck she might even have a place of her own by the end of the week and even if there was any work to be done she could tackle it in the evenings or during the weekends. Apart from anything else it would keep her occupied and her mind off other things, she thought, with a tiny frown.

With the address safely in her bag she made her way to the surgery and began on the list of waiting patients straight away. Luckily it was a fairly routine morning and she finished early whilst Grant was still seeing the remainder of his own list, but her hope that she would be able to have coffee and leave before he finished were doomed as he came in and accepted a cup from Margaret.

Draining her cup hastily she rose to her feet and reached for her bag, purposely avoiding his eye. 'If you'll excuse me, I've a couple of calls to make before I do some errands of my own.' She was half way to the door before his voice halted her in her tracks.

'I'm in something of a hurry myself, Doctor, but if you can spare the time there are one or two things I'd like to discuss . . .' Had she imagined it or was there a definite coolness to his tone? With a barely concealed sigh she turned and felt herself come under a careful scrutiny which unnerved her as his mouth twisted sardonically and she had the distinct impression that he was seeing her in the bath robe, knowing full well that she had had nothing on beneath it. 'I take it you've recovered from your . . . ordeal?'

She stiffened at the obvious sarcasm. 'Perfectly, thank you.'

He nodded, curtly. 'Your car has been fixed at the local garage. I rang them last night. Luckily they're always very obliging. It should have been delivered by now.'

She flushed, caught off guard by the unexpected thoughtfulness. 'Thank you. I'm grateful. As a matter of fact I'd been wondering how I was going to get it seen to. I borrowed Uncle Tom's car this morning.'

'I'll see it gets back to him.'

She waited, willing herself not to look at him and found herself studying a darn in the sleeve of his jacket. It looked ragged, as if he had attempted it himself and she wondered vaguely why the faithful Miss Latimer hadn't obliged. She tore her gaze away from it. 'Well, if that's all . . .'

'No.' He frowned, making an impatient movement with his hand.

'I am in rather a hurry.'

'Really,' the dark brows rose. 'Are we working you too hard?'

'That wasn't what I meant,' she said, sharply. 'I have a call to make and as it happens I also have to go into Foxley on personal business.' She hesitated. 'I want to call in at the estate agents to see if I can find a suitable flat.'

'Aren't you comfortable at Tom's?'

It was really no business of his whether she was or wasn't, she thought and snapped, 'Yes, of course I am. Perfectly comfortable. It's just that I prefer to have a place of my own, somewhere . . .' Blast him, why was he making her feel so uncomfortable?

'Somewhere where you feel safe in your virgin bed? I take it it is a virgin bed?'

She felt the heat scorch her cheeks as she turned abruptly to the door. 'As it happens, I simply decided I would prefer to have a little privacy. I didn't imagine you would have any objections. On the contrary,' her eyes flung a challenge, 'I think the less we see of each other outside the practice, the better, don't you?'

He refused to rise to the bait. 'It's entirely up to you, of course. I was simply thinking that you'll need to find somewhere close to the practice.'

'Oh don't worry about that. I've no intention of being late on duty again, Doctor.' She turned on her heel and marched huffily out into reception before she realised she still didn't know what it was he had wanted to discuss with her.

Margaret Allen was busy re-filing the medical cards as Lee went up to the desk.

'Margaret, I'm going over to see Mrs Jessop. She had a nasty fall and will probably have to be admitted to hospital. After that I shall be in Foxley visiting the estate agents.'

'Oh yes, are you looking for property in the area then, Doctor?'

'A flat, actually. Not too big but somewhere where I can spread a bit, if you know what I mean.'

Margaret Allen grinned. 'I know exactly what

you mean. Dr Jameson's a lovely man and that house of his is huge. Too huge if you ask me for a man on his own, even with Dr Sinclair living there, but a woman likes a place to call her own.'

Lee smiled her relief. 'That's exactly what I mean.'

'I shouldn't think you'll have any trouble, especially not if you see Mr Mowbray personally.'

'Mowbray?'

'Yes, Charles Mowbray. He's the biggest property agent in Foxley and a very nice man.' She glanced sidelong at Lee, taking in the neat cap of curls and the well-cut tweed suit. 'Quite good-looking too as a matter of fact.'

'Yes.' Lee rifled busily in her bag, searching for her car keys. 'At the moment my interests are confined strictly to flat-hunting, but thanks for the information anyway. I'll see Mr Mowbray in person if possible.' She heard the door open behind her as she looked for the elusive keys and Margaret looked up.

'Oh, Dr Sinclair, Miss Latimer is waiting for you in her car. I did explain that you were still with a patient and asked her to come in, but she said she would be perfectly happy where she is and that waiting will give her a nice, healthy appetite.'

In spite of herself, Lee found herself glancing up and was intrigued by the change which spread across his features making him seem briefly relaxed. Obviously Miss Latimer had an amazing effect on him, she thought, as she reached the door.

It opened before she reached it and she almost collided with the figure who came through. The girl was probably in her mid-twenties, tall, attractive and with the kind of thick, dark hair Lee had always secretly envied. Blue-grey eyes passed with smiling but polite uninterest over Lee, then she was laughing and heading straight for Grant's arms.

'Grant, darling, I've just about run out of patience. You owe me a huge meal to make up for letting me down last night, and I warn you I'm ravenous.' She hooked one slender hand through his arm and he was actually laughing down at her.

'And ravishing too.' He bent to kiss her cheek and Lee bent quickly to retrieve her bag which had fallen to the floor as she and the girl had collided. 'Look, give me five minutes and I'll be with you I promise.' His look was suddenly directed at Lee. 'I think we can safely leave things in Dr Forrester's capable hands, for a while at least.'

Lee scowled. She was in no mood for sarcasm. Hunched into her coat, she turned the collar up, gave him a look of disgust and strode out.

So that was Christy Latimer. She was suddenly aware that her hands were gripping the steering wheel too tightly and she forced herself to relax. Why should it matter to her that the woman in Grant Sinclair's life was not just pretty but, if she were honest, quite staggeringly lovely? It's no concern of mine what he does with his spare time and who he spends it with, she told herself firmly. But all the same, a dark cloud of depression seemed to hang over her for no reason for the rest of the morning.

As luck would have it the calls she had to make didn't take too long and an hour spent poring over a large and detailed map of the local area last night, in spite of her weariness, had paid off. She had been able to plan a route which led her conveniently back to town and was even able to find a parking space, miracle of miracles, or perhaps not so much of a miracle since there was a bitingly cold wind and most people with any sense had probably stayed at home.

Locking the Mini she investigated the main shopping area and on impulse found herself buying a beautifully soft sweater in a shade of green she loved. By the time she came out of the shop it was past midday and her stomach was rumbling. She toyed with the idea of finding something to eat and a cup of coffee then, just as the decision was made her eye caught the sign over the local estate agent's office and she decided to suppress a basic need for food in favour of getting the hunt for a flat started as quickly as possible.

Sprinting across the road she let herself thankfully into the warmth of an attractive office. A girl seated at the desk looked up, smiling helpfully. A man stood with his back to her, speaking on the telephone. The voice was pleasant, somehow vaguely familiar, then she dismissed the thought as nonsense and began to explain as concisely as possible to the girl just what she was looking for.

'I'm a doctor so obviously I need something within easy reach of Foxley. At the moment I'm not exactly sure for how long but . . . roughly three months.' The thought flickered rapidly through her head that even if the job didn't last that long she could use the flat as a base for looking for other employment. The girl took a note of the details and was busily flicking her way through a large filing cabinet when the man put down the phone and turned to speak to her. His gaze passed briefly over Lee with a smile of polite interest and she returned the look, then her face lit with instant pleasurable recognition whilst his own changed to one of laughing disbelief.

'You!'

They said it simultaneously and laughed. Lee rose from the chair and found her hands grasped in a firm handshake.

'Well, this is a marvellous surprise!' His eyes were warm as he looked down at her. 'And to think I'd persuaded myself I'd never see my angel of mercy ever again. I have to admit I was disappointed. It's not every day a man finds himself lying in the road and opens his eyes to a beautiful woman ministering to his needs.'

Lee's eyes were bright with laughter. 'I don't make a habit of it.'

'You'll be pleased to hear that neither do I, though I might be persuaded if I thought it would produce you.' His smile was as attractive as his voice. 'Look, how about some coffee? It will give us a chance to talk and you can tell me what you're doing here in this office of all places. By the way, we never did manage to get introduced properly did we?'

Lee chuckled softly. 'The circumstances didn't seem quite right somehow.'

'Well now that they're a little better, I'm Charles Mowbray.'

'Lee Forrester.'

They shook hands again, laughing at the exaggerated formality and Jane Conroy sped away, returning minutes later with coffee as Lee was explaining her predicament.

'So you see, I'd really like somewhere of my own. My room at Dr Jameson's house is very nice but I hate scrambling for the bathroom in the morning, which is why I thought a flat . . .'

'Or a cottage, which would offer even more privacy.'

'Oh yes, but I suppose I'm asking the impossible.'

'As it happens I don't think you are.' He was on his feet, striding across the room and for the first time Lee realised how tall he was. Good-looking too, she thought, as he moved to reach for some papers. He was a little older than she had first imagined, probably in his late thirties. Her glance went to his arm.

'I've just realised I didn't ask how you are now. You don't seem to have suffered any lasting effects after the accident.'

'Oh that.' He flexed the arm carefully. 'It's been painful. The hospital put a nice line of stitches in it and I was kept in overnight because of a mild concussion, but I had no intention of staying around a minute longer than was necessary.'

'I can't say I blame you for that.'

He paused and his gaze looked directly into hers. 'I really am grateful you know. Things might have been much worse.'

She flushed, laughing the suggestion lightly aside. 'I doubt that. In any case Dr Sinclair took over and did most of the work.'

His brows rose. 'You know Grant?'

'Do you?' Her surprise echoed his own.

'Lord yes, from years back.'

'But I didn't realise he was local.'

'No, he isn't. But then, neither am I really. I came up from the south years ago and Grant about three. We'd been at school together as kids, well, not exactly together, I was several years ahead, but we kept in touch vaguely as kids do and he came over a few times and obviously liked what he saw.' There was a slight hesitancy to his voice but it was gone so quickly that Lee put it down to her imagination.

He looked at his watch. 'Look, I've got an idea. These are details of a property which came in just this morning by a piece of luck. I've a feeling you may well be interested. How about looking them over and discussing the possibilities over lunch? I was just going to have some anyway and afterwards, if you like, I can actually take you to see the property.'

Lee couldn't suppress a feeling of excitement that things really seemed to be happening so quickly. She picked up her bag and got to her feet. 'I'd love to.' She couldn't help but feel flattered by the look of surprised relief which crossed his face as he grinned.

'Fine. I know a super pub where they do hot meals as well as snacks.'

'It sounds marvellous.'

And it was. Replete after a superb meal Lee sat back drinking coffee and thinking how easy Charles Mowbray was to get along with. She might have known him for years. Refusing more coffee she sat studying the details he had given her of a cottage which sounded almost too good to be true.

'I can hardly believe it, and the rent is so reasonable too. Are you sure there isn't a catch?' She looked at him. 'I mean it has everything, bathroom, kitchen, telephone, garden. Is it falling down a cliff or something equally diabolical?'

He laughed and she was vaguely conscious of his arm resting along the seat behind her. 'I assure you it isn't. We don't have cliffs in this part of the world. Seriously though, it's in superb condition and the owner is prepared to let for anything up to six months with an option for longer if necessary.' His brown eyes studied her seriously. 'I'm rather hoping you'll want to take up that option if you don't mind my saying so.'

Lee felt herself blush. 'No, of course I don't mind. I rather like the idea myself, if it's all you say it is. It's just that my plans are a little uncertain . . .'

'Yes of course, I understand that. Still, what do you think?'

She glanced at the papers again. 'Well, what can I say, apart from the fact that I'd love to see it even if I still can't believe it's true.'

His mouth contorted. 'I suppose I'd better come clean. As a matter of fact I know the owner. She happens to be an aunt of mine and she's just flown off to Australia on an indefinite visit to her sister. They haven't met for about fifty years and I rather suspect all the catching up they'll have to do will take another fifty.' He laughed. 'She asked me to take care of things for her and you just happened to come along at precisely the right time. Speaking personally I couldn't have asked for anyone I'd rather have as a tenant. You are thinking seriously about it, aren't you?'

'More and more so every minute,' Lee laughed, breathlessly. 'But how soon would I be able to move in, if it does happen to be what I'm looking for?'

'Just as soon as you like. Tomorrow if you want to, once you've looked the place over, but I'm sure you'll love it.'

And he was right, Lee thought, as she returned to stand in the sitting room of the cottage and looked round at the large open fireplace, the comfortable furnishings and the gleaming copper ornaments scattered so lovingly around the room. She sighed happily.

'I'll take it of course. It's perfect and I'll do as you say and move in tomorrow after surgery. I don't have many things—one car load should do it easily and anything else I need I can always buy.'

'That's what I like, a girl who knows her own mind. I'll give you a hand if you like.'

It needed only the briefest reflection to decide that she did like. It was rather nice to be able to talk to someone outside the practice and about things other than medicine, and apart from that, it took her mind off Grant Sinclair. 'Yes I would. I'd be grateful.'

Charles grinned and stuck his hands in his pockets. 'I charge rather high rates I'm afraid. At least a cup of coffee and a glass of whisky if it runs into overtime.'

'Well that sounds reasonable.' She giggled and followed him out to the car, pausing beside him to turn and take a long, backward glance at what was to be her home for at least the next three months, all being well.

Returning to the office it took scarcely any time at all to sign the necessary papers, then the keys were in her hand.

'Welcome to your new home,' Charles murmured, retaining his hold on them for a moment longer than necessary so that his fingers brushed against hers.

DOCTORS IN DISPUTE

Lee smiled awkwardly, not unaware that things might be moving rather more quickly where Charles Mowbray was concerned than she was ready for, or was she complicating things unnecessarily in her own mind? He was a very nice, attractive man and they were both free agents. She said briskly, 'Yes, well it will be, as soon as I get myself organised. I'd better go. There are a million things to do before I move in tomorrow.'

With the keys jingling in her pocket she went back to Uncle Tom's and began to pack.

CHAPTER SIX

'So you really are moving?'

Lee looked up, frowning, from the letter she had just finished writing. The last patient had gone and she had been so busy tidying up a few loose ends that she hadn't even heard Grant come into her room. Now a groove of annoyance edged its way into her features.

'That's right. I've managed to find a cottage.'

'Really? Quick work.'

There was a note of sarcasm in his voice which she chose to ignore. Getting to her feet she found herself deliberately finding things to do rather than sit there being studied. She drew back the curtains from round the examination couch, spending more time than was necessary on arranging the folds.

'I suppose it was. It was quite a coincidence really. The agency I went to is run by Charles Mowbray, the man who had the accident.' It was her turn to meet his gaze directly now and she felt swift pleasure in the fact that he had the grace to look vaguely discomfited. 'I gather you and he know each other.'

'We were at school together. I don't know that that's knowing.'

'Yes, he told me.'

'It's a small world.'

Too small, she thought, acidly. 'The cottage belongs to his aunt. She went to Australia last week and Charles was looking for someone to take over the tenancy.'

'How very convenient,' he drawled. 'You'll be neighbours. Lucky old Charles.'

She hadn't been aware that she had used Charles' name until then. It had slipped out quite innocently, but then, why not, she thought, crossly. They had lunched together and under the circumstances formality would have been ridiculous. Besides, what she did with her private life was nothing to do with Grant Sinclair, provided it didn't interfere with her work and there was no chance of that. She smiled sweetly. 'Yes, he thinks so too. As a matter of fact he's coming over this evening after surgery to help me move my things.' She gathered up the case notes, half hoping he would take the hint and leave. Infuriatingly he leaned nonchalantly against the desk, watching her with maddening inscrutability.

'You certainly don't waste any time, do you? Are you always so certain about what you want?'

There was something in the way he asked the question that made her head jerk up, green eyes uncompromising. 'I try to be, Doctor. I'm sorry if that doesn't happen to meet with your approval.'

The dark brows narrowed. 'I didn't say I disapproved. What ever gave you the idea that I would?'

Lee gritted her teeth, looking swiftly away. She couldn't imagine why she should have thought it. In fact the more she got to know about Grant Sinclair the more she realised that he was a man with very definite views about what he wanted and with the realisation came the uneasy thought that he would use any means to get it.

She slammed the drawer of the filing cabinet. 'Did you want me for something specific, or was this merely a social call?'

'Oh, it was definitely something specific.'

Lee felt her colour rise. 'Then would you mind coming to the point. I'd like to get away as early as possible.'

'Far be it from me to detain you then,' he said, dryly. 'I just wanted to say that I have to attend a conference tomorrow and I'm not sure what time I'll be back. It may be late.' He frowned. 'I suppose I could cancel but it's pretty important.'

Lee stiffened. 'I really see no reason for you to do that. I'm perfectly capable of coping here for one day. I doubt if the practice is going to grind to a complete halt even in your absence, Doctor.' She saw by the sudden tightening of his mouth that she had scored a hit, but for some reason the thought failed to give the pleasure she had expected. There was just something about him that put her immediately on the defensive and she didn't like it. It left her feeling uneasy.

'I suppose I'll have to take your word for it.' He strode to the door, his face like thunder. 'By the way, give my regards to Charles.'

She didn't answer and minutes later heard his car drive away. No doubt the lovely Miss Latimer will soothe his ruffled feathers, she thought, and promptly put him from her mind as she began planning what she had to take over to the cottage.

A fire was burning cheerfully in the hearth as Lee dumped her suitcase and Charles followed her in from the car with a box of groceries.

'I got Mrs Slater to pop in and put a match to the fire,' he said as she expressed her appreciation. 'She's agreed to come in twice a week to dust and generally make sure the place is kept clean, and aired but I'm sure if you want her to she'll fit in with any arrangement you care to make. I don't suppose you get much time.'

'Well it would certainly be useful and nice to come home to a warm fire in the evenings, at least during this cold spell. If you're sure she won't mind?'

'Actually I've already suggested it to her, tentatively, and she'll be delighted. Now, if you'll tell me where you want these things I'll oblige.'

He carried the large suitcase upstairs leaving Lee to stow away the groceries in the refrigerator and various cupboards, and when she returned to the sitting room he greeted her with two glasses of wine.

'I hope you don't mind. I brought this with me, just by way of a little celebration.'

She felt inordinately touched by the gesture and smiled as she accepted one of the glasses. 'Why should I mind? I think it's a lovely idea even though I can still scarcely believe it's all happened and so quickly too.'

He made a mocking little bow and sat beside her on the large, comfortable couch. 'Our policy is to please and we lay strong emphasis on the personal touch.'

'You mean you give this kind of service to all your clients?'

'Well no, only those we like and want to get to know better and I have to admit that I hope this is just the start of a long and beautiful friendship, you know that, don't you, Lee?'

Feeling suddenly awkward she took a long sip of the wine and stared down into the glass. 'Don't let's rush anything, Charles. I'd like very much for us to be friends too, but let's take it one day at a time. Besides,' she laughed lightly, easing the sudden tension, 'there's a grave danger that you might be mistaking gratitude for something else. Just because I happened to come along in your hour of need . . .'

'I don't think there's any danger of my making that kind of mistake.' He leaned towards her and brushed his lips lightly against her cheek. She made no attempt to prevent it but she got to her feet the moment he released her and he followed suit, taking the glass from her and putting it on the table with his own.

'You're tired.'

She blinked, suddenly realising that she was, and was grateful to him for understanding and respecting her wariness without referring to it. 'It's been a long day and a very eventful one, thanks to you, but I still have to be up at the crack of dawn.' She looked up at him. 'Do you mind awfully?'

'Why should I mind.' With an easy gesture he put his hands on her shoulders and smiled. 'Perhaps I could see you tomorrow. We could go for a meal somewhere.'

It sounded nice, then she grimaced. 'Oh I can't, not tomorrow. I just remembered, Grant is away at a conference, in London I think, and he's not sure what time he'll be back so I have to cover.'

'Oh well, can't be helped.' He brushed her cheek lightly with his fingers then put her firmly from him with a rueful sigh. 'I think you're right, it is time I went but I'll call you.'

'Yes, do.' She realised that she actually meant it. It would be nice to go out with Charles, but the idea had already slipped from her mind by the time she had had a quick shower and finally slipped between the sheets to dream of Charles, except that every time she found herself in his arms and looked up at his face, the features somehow disturbingly became those of Grant Sinclair.

CHAPTER SEVEN

LEE hummed softly to herself as she drove to the surgery the following morning. It had stopped snowing and the sun was shining palely, melting the crystal drops hanging from the trees. It was even possible to summon a belief that spring was on the way. Or, if she was more honest with herself, her good mood probably owed more to the fact that Grant was away. Whatever the reason she wasn't going to have it spoilt by thinking about him and she walked into Reception smiling as she unfastened her coat.

'Morning, Margaret.'

'Good morning, Doctor. You're nice and early.' She handed Lee the mail which had already been sorted and Lee flicked through it ruefully, recognising the inevitable promotions which detailed the very latest in new drugs and medical care.

'It looks as if I'm going to be kept pretty busy doing some late night reading,' she said.

'And there's a rep to see you as well, Doctor.' Margaret nodded in the direction of the waiting room. 'He's been there for half an hour. Would you like to see him now?'

'Are we very busy?'

Margaret consulted the list. 'Not too bad at the

moment but building up steadily.'

'Well in that case if he just wants to show me some follow-up material on something he's already discussed with Dr Sinclair I'll see him. If it's something that needs more time and my undivided attention will you ask him if he would prefer to hang on and see me later or come back before this evening's surgery.'

'I'll do that, Doctor.' Margaret nodded briskly and reached for the telephone as it rang, covering the mouthpiece as she said, 'I was going to ask about the cottage but I think it had better wait. Oh and Dr Sinclair left this note before he went off to London this morning.' She handed Lee an envelope.

'He's already been in?'

'So I gather. It must have been very early. I found that on my desk when I arrived.'

'Setting us all a good example, no doubt,' Lee muttered as she took the letter with her into the surgery. Well, she refused to be impressed. It was probably a long list of instructions, strongly backed with the implication that she couldn't do her job unless properly supervised. 'You can just sit there and wait until I'm ready for you, Doctor.' She propped the letter up on her desk and rang the bell for her first patient who turned out to be plural, two very spotty, very fractious five-year-old twins who promptly proceeded to empty a jar of throat spatulas all over the floor, unhindered in their efforts by their exhausted-looking mother who clearly welcomed any cessation in their demands upon herself.

'They fair wear me out, Doctor,' she admitted, rifling in a voluminous shopping bag from which she produced two bars of chocolate. They were leapt upon eagerly whilst Lee tried hard not to flinch. 'I can't turn my back for five minutes without they're up to something.'

Lee could believe it as she rescued her prescription pad from a sticky hand and sent the mother and her offspring happily on their way before her next patient came in.

It was a routine surgery followed by half an hour's in-depth discussion with the sales representative who left her with samples of a new product and yet more informative literature. It was only as she added it to the growing pile in her briefcase that she remembered Grant Sinclair's letter and grudgingly tore the envelope open.

To her surprise it contained not the expected list but a note written in a large, untidy scrawl. It was brief almost to the point of being curt.

'I thought you'd be pleased to hear that Mrs Cox and her baby are doing well. Mr Cox telephoned to say they have decided to name her after you, if you have no objections that is. I took the liberty of saying I was sure it would be all right. Oh and perhaps I should also take this opportunity to add my own thanks. Events didn't make it seem entirely appropriate at the time!'

It was grudging, yet for some inexplicable reason the words sent a ridiculous surge of pleasure flooding through her. It vanished however as she read on: *'I hope to be back this evening, but should you need to contact me urgently you can reach me at . . .'* Her fingers closed angrily over the telephone number.

'Don't hurry back on my account, Dr Sinclair. You may be unhappy to hear that we are managing perfectly well without you.'

It was a luxury to be able to finish the morning calls and go back to the cottage where Mrs Slater had left a superb casserole in the oven. It smelled delicious and tasted even better and Lee found herself eating ravenously as she balanced a tray on her knees and skimmed quickly through the morning paper before making a start on the mountain of jobs she had promised herself she would do.

On the way back from town she had stopped at the local florists and now she spent some time arranging to best advantage the half dozen plants she had tempted herself into buying. That done, she unwrapped the new, delicate tea service which had also caught her eye in one of the large stores. There was an abundance of crockery left by the cottage's owner but somehow Lee suspected they were all treasured pieces and the thought that any of them might get broken was more than she cared to contemplate. In any case it was nice to have something of her very own. It was a bit like setting up home, she thought wryly, except that there was no man around to enjoy her efforts and somehow, when she tried to conjure up an image of Charles sitting comfortably in one of the large arm chairs, the picture didn't seem to fit.

'I could make it fit,' she thought, with a flash of irritation. There would be something very nice, very comforting about coming home in the evening to a warm fireside and a man like Charles. 'I just need time to get used to the idea.' She would have to take him up on that offer of a meal sometime.

The phone rang and she almost laughed aloud as Charles's voice spoke persuasively in her ear.

'I know you're busy tonight but I've had an invitation to a dinner party in a few days' time and you're included, if you'd like it that is.'

Suppressing a giggle she said, with genuine warmth, 'That sounds lovely.'

There was a momentary silence at the other end of the phone, then he said, 'I say, are you all right?'

She could imagine him frowning. 'Yes, I'm fine, why?' Perhaps something in her voice had given away the fact that she had been assessing him as possible husband material.

'Nothing. You just sound a bit odd, that's all.'

'Really?' she said, brightly. 'I think I'm going in for a bit of a cold.'

'Oh, well as long as that's all it is.' His voice sounded a little husky. Perhaps he was going in for a cold too. 'I still think you need someone to take you in hand.' He rang off, chuckling, before she had time to answer and she found herself smiling as she made her way upstairs and began to survey the mound of unpacking still left from yesterday. By the time she had hung up all her clothes in the wardrobe it was already quite dark and there was just time to make herself a cup of coffee and a sandwich before going back to Foxley to take the evening surgery.

There was still no word from Grant by the time she had finished. 'Not that I'm altogether surprised,' Margaret confessed. 'You know what these conferences are. I've known them to run on quite late. Still, it's lucky he has you here to take over. I know how important this particular one was to him. He's been talking about attending for months and then when Dr Jameson had his heart attack . . . well, it looked for a while as if he wouldn't be able to make it after all, and that would have been a shame especially as the organisers have been trying for a long time to persuade him to give a lecture.'

Lee found herself grudgingly curious. 'You mean he's actually speaking?'

'Oh yes. In fact I think he's the main speaker, but then he was probably one of the best authorities in the country on renal disease until he decided to give it all up. Frankly I think it seems an awful shame. Such a waste.'

Lee was aware that she was standing open-mouthed, staring. 'Grant Sinclair, an expert on renal disease.' Suddenly she felt quite cold. 'Are you sure? You couldn't possibly have mistaken him for someone else?'

'Good heavens, no.' Margaret sealed the last envelope for the post. 'I thought you knew.'

'No, no I didn't.' She shook her head. 'But then, I suppose we haven't really had much chance to talk.'

'I don't suppose he thought it necessary. I mean, since he decided to give up that side of medicine and come here. I only found out by accident, more or less, because several letters were delivered here for him after he first arrived . . .'

Lee knew she shouldn't encourage the receptionist to gossip but suddenly she desperately needed to know more about this other side of Grant Sinclair's character.

'But what made him give it up, and why come here, to a small place like Foxley?'

The telephone rang, breaking the moment for confidences, even had there been any. Margaret Allen reached for it, silencing its persistence. 'I don't know. He didn't ever seem inclined to talk about it. Hullo . . . yes, Dr Sinclair's surgery. No, I'm sorry, Dr Sinclair isn't in this evening. I'll ask Dr Forrester to call.' She glanced at Lee who nodded. 'Fine, Doctor will be out as soon as possible then, Mrs Stevens. No, I can't say exactly when. Doctor has a couple of other calls to make but it won't be late.'

Lee went back to the surgery to collect her bag and check that its contents were ready for any emergency, but somehow instead she found herself sitting at the desk thinking about Grant Sinclair until, with a sigh of frustration she realised she was wasting her time. Grant Sinclair was an enigma and she didn't like enigmas, and apart from anything else she wasn't going to be in Foxley long enough to try and unravel the mystery.

All the same, lying awake that night, staring up at the low, uneven ceiling, she found her thoughts drifting back to the subject. Why would anyone, doing such valuable work, someone who had obviously earned a well-deserved reputation for himself if Margaret Allen's gossip was true, suddenly give it all up to become a GP in a small backwater like Foxley?

She sighed, tossing restlessly as the more she pondered on it the more the answers seemed to evade her. Glancing at the clock she lay for a minute, her arm flung across her eyes. She should be getting some sleep, she thought, irritably, not lying here trying to solve the mystery of Grant Sinclair.

It was one o'clock. She wondered what time he had got back and with a stifled moan of impatience flung back the covers, reached for a dressing gown and padded, shivering, down to the kitchen to make herself a warm milk drink, sitting at the table, stifling her yawns as the milk heated.

It helped. She must have finally drifted off into a heavy sleep about half an hour later so that when she woke suddenly to the loud shrilling of the telephone and gazed disbelievingly at the clock which now said two-thirty, she felt shaky and drugged as she spoke into the receiver. 'Dr Forrester.'

Minutes later she was struggling back into her

clothes as the kettle boiled and she gulped scalding black coffee to wake herself up. Her bag was ready beside her coat. Barely flicking a comb through her hair she went out to the car, gasping as a wave of cold air hit her.

As she drove she reflected that Grant was obviously not back after all, since her caller had tried his telephone number and been directed instead to call her. The road was icy and it needed all her powers of concentration to keep the car steady. What if he had had an accident? The thought flashed briefly through her mind and her hand tightened spasmodically against the wheel.

She pulled up and looked at the house where lights blazed. Walking up the path she briefly had time to notice that the sky was clear and full of stars before the door was opened and a figure drew her anxiously into the house, someone who had obviously been waiting for the sound of the car.

'Oh, Doctor, thank God you've come. I didn't know what to do.'

Lee gently ushered the woman inside. 'Where is your husband, Mrs Anderson? Upstairs?'

'No,' her lips quivered. 'That's it you see,' she led Lee towards the kitchen, 'he must have got up to make some tea without me hearing him. Ted often does that. He's not a very good sleeper.'

Lee walked into the kitchen, took one look at the man lying on the floor and went quickly towards him, dropping her bag onto the table. His face was greyish blue and her hand felt rapidly for a pulse.

'It's a heart attack, isn't it, Doctor.' Tears flooded into the woman's eyes as Lee nodded.

'I'm afraid so, though at this stage it's impossible to tell how bad it is.'

A shuddering sigh escaped the woman's lips. 'I wouldn't have known. He might have lain there all night if he hadn't knocked the jug over as he fell. It was the crash that woke me you see. He . . . he said it was only indigestion but I could see it wasn't. I told him I was going to call an ambulance but he started getting fidgety and cross and then . . . well I said I was going to call the doctor and just after I did . . . this happened.'

Lee was on her feet scarcely hearing what the distraught woman was saying. 'Do you have a telephone, Mrs Anderson?'

'What . . . oh yes, Doctor.'

'Fine, I'm going to get that ambulance here now. It should take a few minutes. In the meantime if you want to pack a few of your husband's things into a bag.'

'I want to go with him, Doctor.'

Lee nodded gently. 'Yes, of course you do.' She scanned the small figure still clad in night-clothes. 'If the ambulance gets here before you're ready I think it would be as well if they get your husband off to the hospital where he can be looked after as soon as possible, but I'll drive you there myself.'

As she was speaking she was already dialling the number of the local hospital and as she replaced the receiver she breathed an inward sigh of relief. At least help was on its way, but it was still going to be a long struggle for Ted Anderson.

It was four o'clock before she finally got back to the cottage to find that the fire had gone out and that all thoughts of sleep had left her. After a few years she would probably get used to it, take it all in her stride, but at this moment she felt too keyed up, too depressed, thinking of the elderly couple, to be able simply to climb back into bed and sleep.

Funnily enough, she had an appetite and having thrown a large log into the still faintly glowing ashes she went into the kitchen, made herself a sandwich and carried it back to the sitting room. The pangs of hunger satisfied she sat staring into the fire listening to the crackle of the wood and wishing Grant were here. 'I must be over-tired,' she muttered to herself, resting her head back on the large, soft cushion. The last person she wanted to see was Grant Sinclair. All the same his shadowy figure haunted her dreams as, warmed by the glow of the fire, she drifted into an uneasy sleep.

It was some time later that she woke again, this time feeling cross and irritable. She hadn't meant to fall asleep on the sofa and having done so felt worse. Shivering she glanced at her watch. Half past five. 'Oh no. Well it's hardly worth going to bed now,' she muttered.

Flinging off her clothes she took a quick shower, dressed in a soft, woollen skirt and jumper and made herself some more coffee. Scanning her reflection in the mirror she noted the dark shadows under her eyes and reproved herself for not having had the sense to try and make herself get to bed and sleep properly. It was just as well Grant was going to be back to take morning surgery.

The sky was just beginning to brighten as she pulled back the curtains, and there was actually some faint promise of a fine day. Whether it was that or the gritty feeling in her eyes she decided on the spur of the moment to take a short, brisk walk. It would get some air into her lungs and probably have more effect than half a dozen cups of coffee, she thought.

Minutes later, clad in a warm sheepskin jacket, she was striding out in comfortable, country brogues, along the lanes looking for signs that perhaps at last winter might be over. She began to visualise the countryside as it would be a few weeks from now, when everything was fresh and green, the woods filled with bluebells and the sun glistening on the large reservoir not many miles away. She felt a sudden tightening in her chest as she realised that she would probably never see it like that.

By the time she had returned from her walk twenty minutes later, her feeling of mild depression had gone. She felt cold but refreshed and was actually enjoying a breakfast of scrambled eggs on toast when the phone rang, shattering the peace and quiet. Reaching for it she swallowed hard on a piece of toast.

'Dr Forrester speaking.'

'Well thank God for that,' Grant Sinclair's voice

intruded angrily upon her newly restored good humour. 'Where the devil have you been? I've been trying for the best part of the night to get hold of you. I suppose you've been out wining and dining and don't give a hang about the patients.'

Lee felt the anger flood into her throat at the injustice of the words. Her cheeks were white as she tried to speak. 'No, Doctor. As it happens . . .'

'Spare me the details, for pity's sake,' his voice cut in, icily, 'I'm not interested and I don't have the time. I'm in a call box and I don't have any change.'

'A call box? But why, where . . . ?'

'I'm trying to explain, if you'll just give me a chance. The conference went on much later than expected. I tried to get away but couldn't. You know how these things are?' She didn't but could imagine. 'Then when I eventually made my escape there was a heavy snow fall and I had to pull in at one of the motorway service areas and that's where I am now.' His voice tightened. 'I'm sorry, but you'll just have to take this morning's surgery. With a bit of luck I may get there in time to take over. The weather has improved slightly but it's still going to take me a while to get to Foxley.'

Lee heard her own voice sounding strangely strangled. 'But I've only . . .'

His voice cut in sharply again. 'Look, I don't have time to argue. I haven't had any sleep, I need some coffee, some breakfast and a shave. I'm sorry, Doctor, if your work happens to conflict with the needs of your social life, but that's the way it goes.'

She had just opened her mouth to fling an angry response at him when the receiver snapped noisily into place and he was gone, leaving her shaking with fury. 'How dare he?' she muttered through clenched teeth as she made a hurried grab for her bag, angrily surveyed the ruins of her breakfast and rushed to spend a few minutes applying a delicate film of make-up to her face in an attempt to blot out any evidence of her night's 'orgy'.

She was still seething as she locked the door and hurried out yet again to the car. And now if she didn't hurry she was going to be late, which would, no doubt, please him even more!

CHAPTER EIGHT

'It's pretty full in there, I'm afraid.' Margaret nodded in the direction of the waiting room. 'And all yours, I hate to tell you. Dr Sinclair isn't back yet.'

Lee found it difficult to keep the note of iciness from her voice. 'No, he phoned me, from a motorway service station somewhere. He was just about to have breakfast.' She knew she hadn't altogether succeeded as curiosity briefly widened the older woman's eyes. 'Well, I suppose it seemed the most sensible thing to do, knowing that no one would be manning the phone here until you arrived, and it's just as well or I'd never have made it in time.' She hid a yawn behind her hand. 'I don't know what's the matter with me this morning. I can't seem to get going.'

'Yes, you look a bit peaky. I hope you're not going in for a dose of this 'flu that seems to be going around.'

'Oh no, I'm fine really. I just didn't sleep too well and then I was called out to Mr Anderson. He had a heart attack. I managed to get him to hospital but it's going to be touch and go for a while.'

'The poor man.'

'Mm, his poor wife too. I'll write up the notes and

let you have them later. I'll probably phone the hospital too. I'd like to know how he's doing.' She picked up the pile of cards. 'I shouldn't think his wife got any sleep either. I drove her to the hospital myself so that she could be with him.'

'No wonder you're tired. I tell you what, I'll go and make you a nice strong cup of coffee before you start.'

'Now that sounds like a very good idea.' Lee smiled wearily. 'And if you could rustle up a couple of aspirins too . . .'

'I should think I can manage that.' She hurried away to the small kitchen and minutes later put a cup of steaming hot coffee and two tablets on Lee's desk. 'You drink up and I'll wheel the first patient in in a couple of minutes.'

'Bless you. Let's just hope they're all straightforward, though having said that I dare say every one will have complications of one sort or another.'

It was a relief to find herself proved wrong for once, however, and she eyed the diminishing pile of cards with satisfaction as she rang the bell for the next patient and a young woman came in with a small child who looked decidedly feverish and was crying lethargically.

Lee questioned the mother whilst making a gentle examination of the child who was two years old.

'I can't understand it, Doctor. Susie's not a child who complains, but she's bright and when she says she's got a headache I know she means it.'

Lee nodded. 'Yes, I can see she has, and quite a nasty one too by the look of her.' She took a fever-strip from her drawer and pressed it to the child's forehead. The temperature was definitely raised but there was no evidence of an inflamed throat. 'Has she complained of a tummy ache?'

The woman frowned. 'No, but funnily enough she has been sick and she seems to have been bumping into things, as if she's giddy, you know what I mean, although one minute she's like this and the next minute right as rain.'

'Ah,' Lee smiled and drew the child towards her, sitting her comfortably on her knee. 'Well suppose we take a quick look in your ears, Susie, and let's see what's going on in there, shall we? Has she had a cold, Mrs Reynolds?'

'Well yes, as a matter of fact she has, Doctor. A couple of weeks ago. It was quite a heavy one but she seemed to get over it, more or less.'

Lee made a gentle examination of the child's ears and then listened to her chest, confirming the suspicion which had gradually begun to form in her mind. Passing the child back to her mother she wrote out a prescription. 'I'm going to give you some Stemetil, Mrs Reynolds. You'll find it will help the sickness and the balance problem. In fact the two are connected. It's a bit like sea-sickness you see, because Susie has labyrinthitis.'

'Labyrinthitis. I've never heard of it, Doctor.'

'No, it's quite rare in children as young as Susie. What happens is that her ears have become affected by the heavy cold and it's because of that that her balance is affected and that causes her to be sick. But as I say, this medicine should help and I'm going to give you an antibiotic too because her chest is still quite rattly. I'm sure you'll see a rapid improvement over the next few days. She may seem a bit drowsy, but sleep is probably the best thing for her just now, and do be sure she takes all the antibiotic won't you? So often people take half the bottle and then because they feel better don't finish it, then they wonder why in a few weeks' time they feel worse than ever.'

Mrs Reynolds got to her feet clutching the prescription with a smile of relief. 'Don't worry, Doctor, I'll see she takes it all. It will be such a relief to have her back to normal again. I know I complain when she's noisy but I'd much rather have her that way than like this.'

It was a cry echoed by so many mothers and Lee smiled. She would never understand the feeling of guilt built up by so many women simply because they found it almost impossible to cope twenty-four hours a day, fifty-two weeks of the year with a boisterous child without occasionally losing their tempers.

She had just seen the last patient and was looking forward to her coffee break when someone tapped at the door and came in. She frowned because she was certain Margaret had said there were no more patients and the frown deepened as she looked up and saw Grant. She realised then that the car she had heard pulling noisily into the drive must have been his.

She rose to her feet, glancing witheringly in his direction. His comments earlier on the phone still rankled and she said, stiffly, 'Surgery is over, Doctor, entirely without mishap you'll be pleased to hear. I assume that is why you're here. To check up on my competence.'

Immediately she wished the words unsaid as he drew a hand wearily across his forehead, then his face tightened. 'No, as a matter of fact that isn't why I came. I can assure you that if I'd had any doubts at all about your competence I wouldn't have left you to cope here.'

Lee felt her colour rise. 'I may be obtuse, Doctor, but I understand that that was exactly what you implied, or was it simply my morals that were in doubt?'

'Oh that.' His brows drew together in a frown.

'That precisely, Doctor.'

'Look,' his hand thudded against the desk, 'I'm bloody tired and I was worried sick about getting held up. For crying out loud, I scarcely even remember what I said.' He brushed a hand through his hair, leaving a tuft standing on end. It made him look boyish and oddly vulnerable and for one crazy moment she had to stifle an impulse to go to him and smooth it down. She drew herself up, sharply.

'Well I remember perfectly, and I assure you I am not in the habit of being spoken to in such a manner '

'Not even when it's justified?' He looked at her with slow deliberation and she felt her breathing deepen.

'Off duty, Doctor, I am free to do as I please, see whom I please. I do not need your permission. My personal life has nothing whatsoever to do with you.'

'I agree. Provided it doesn't interfere with your work.' His voice was grimly determined but her own was equally so as she faced him, aware of the hot colour scorching her cheeks.

'The things you said were *not* justified, and I very much resent the implication that they were. I have given you no reason to suppose that I would allow anything to interfere with my job here.'

There was a short silence during which his face clouded before he said, curtly, 'You're right. What you do with your life is none of my business.' His mouth tightened. 'As for what I said . . . I owe you an apology. I know it was completely unjustified and the fact that I was tired was no excuse.'

Shock held her rigid and speechless for a minute. 'You know?'

His hand rose in a dismissive gesture. 'I spoke to Margaret. I gather you were called out.'

'As I would have explained, if you had given me the chance.' She was glad he had the grace to look shame-faced.

'I'm sorry. The conference was hard going and I was genuinely worried about the work load I've thrust upon you since you came here.'

Incredibly, she found her defences crumbling. She even managed to smile. 'I thought that was the idea, that I should shoulder some of the burden.'

'Tom's idea, not mine.'

'Aren't you carrying this pig-headedness a bit far?' she flashed angrily. His mouth, a taut line of weariness relaxed suddenly.

'I've got a great idea, why don't we call a truce? It would be a lot less wearing. You're right. I've been unreasonable, but these past few months haven't been particularly easy.'

'I can understand that. I'm as concerned about Tom as you are, but it isn't going to help if we're constantly at loggerheads, is it?'

He sat on the edge of the desk, watching as she tidied it without really thinking what she was doing. His nearness was making her uneasy, then suddenly his hand came down over hers, halting its movements, sending her gaze flying up to meet his.

'Truce?' he repeated. 'And can't we make a start by you calling me Grant. It is my name, you know.'

Her breath caught in her throat as she laughed. 'Well, I suppose it's worth a try, Grant.' His face was close and almost before she knew what was happening he had drawn her unresistingly towards him. She was in the circle of his arms as he rose to his feet, the desk pressing into her back. For a second she stared at him, then his mouth came down, brushing lightly against her lips at first and then, as she drew a quivering breath, the pressure deepened until it became demanding and she felt herself respond with a desperate urgency which left her trembling violently. It was utterly crazy, she told herself. He had said truce, not total surrender. Her hands moved up to his neck and his arms tightened like a steel band around her. She had been kissed before, but never like this, and she heard her own swift gasp of shock as the contact renewed all the previous fire of that other encounter.

The sound of the phone ringing behind her brought her back to reality. Grant cursed under his breath as she tried to move.

'Let it ring.' His lips drew her own back but with the strident ringing common sense returned rapidly and she pushed him gently away, trying to steady her breathing. What if someone had come in? Her hands went to her flushed cheeks.

'I can't. It might be urgent.' She groped behind her for the phone, fumbling with the receiver as Grant's face followed her own until she deliberately tilted her head away out of his reach and said breathlessly, 'Dr Forrester.'

Grant murmured wickedly against her ear, 'It's Lee. We're dropping the formality, remember?'

In desperation she pushed him away as the voice said, 'Hullo, Lee, I hope I haven't called at a bad moment. I waited until I thought surgery would be over.'

The laughter slid from her eyes, taking with it some of the giddy sense of elation. 'Ch . . .

Charles. Hullo, no it's fine. Surgery finished about ten minutes ago.'

'Oh well, in that case it's lucky I caught you.'

She was aware of Grant straightening up, his face suddenly a frozen mask. She wanted to draw him back, regain the moment. Her voice shook. 'Yes, it is.' Her eyes followed him to the door, imploring him to wait, but Charles' voice held her relentlessly.

'I just called to remind you about tonight. I'll pick you up about eight if that's all right?'

'Tonight.' Her brain worked feverishly and her spirits sank. Of course. He was taking her out to dinner. 'Yes, that will be fine. I'll be ready.' What she wanted to say was 'Look, I've changed my mind.' But she dropped the receiver back into place and turned to see Grant standing at the door, his face suddenly like that of a stranger again. The kiss might never have been, except that her mouth still burned from the pressure of his mouth.

'I'd better get going. Obviously you have important business elsewhere.'

'Grant.' Her voice dragged the name out but her feet felt too leaden to go after him. 'I arranged several days ago to go out to dinner with Charles tonight.' She didn't know why she offered the explanation. The words sounded garbled even to her own ears but he seemed totally indifferent.

'You're right, what you do outside of this office is none of my business.' His voice sounded so cold, so unfamiliar, that she flinched. 'Oh by the way, I shall be taking surgery tonight so enjoy yourself and don't forget to give my regards to Charles.'

The door slammed to a close and she was shocked to find her eyes filling with tears. 'Damn,' she swore under her breath, 'damn, damn, damn.' Then she shook herself mentally. After all, wasn't she reading far too much into one simple kiss which, judging from Grant's expression as he had walked out of the door, obviously hadn't meant anything to him. Except, she told herself, that it hadn't been a simple kiss because no simple kiss left you feeling as if not only your mouth but your entire body were on fire.

CHAPTER NINE

IT WAS ludicrous, she thought as she drove back to the cottage later, to find herself actually resenting a whole afternoon of unplanned idleness. It was a luxury she had been promising herself ever since her arrival at Foxley but now that the miracle had happened, somehow the prospect of spending several hours on household chores had definitely lost its charm.

Sitting in the neat little kitchen waiting for some soup to heat she toyed briefly with the idea of ringing Charles and putting off their date, pleading a dose of 'flu. She did have a headache and she was slightly flushed, but on reflection it seemed cowardly to use something that was purely mental rather than physical as an excuse. And in any case an evening with Charles would probably be quite enjoyable. At least it would be uncomplicated she decided, and, having eaten her soup, went up to the low-ceilinged bedroom to scan the contents of her wardrobe and decide what she should wear.

The results provided a minor crisis. When she had packed to come to Foxley it had been with the sole notion that she was going to be working hard for a few weeks and then returning home. Thoughts of any kind of social life had been vague and now that she looked at the one 'dressy' dress she had brought with her, holding the autumn-coloured silk in front of her, it seemed not only dull but old-fashioned.

'Or is it just me?' she spoke to her reflection. 'What I really need is a new image, but am I likely to find it in Foxley I ask myself?'

It was a spur of the moment decision to drive not to the village but into Leicester, several miles away, where she managed to get her hair styled and shampooed. She emerged from the salon with blonde curls flicked into a shining, gamine style which boosted her morale and turned the hunt for a new dress into a necessity rather than a chore. Without knowing exactly what she was looking for she found it, gasped a little at the price, but came out of the shop clutching a bag which contained a beautifully cut dress in a delicate shade of palest greeny-blue, with a high collar and full skirts which swished beautifully as she moved.

Purchase made she drove to see Tom Jameson having promised her father she would send a report on his progress and put his mind at rest. When she arrived at the house, however, the door was opened by Mrs Dawson whose anxious face cleared with relief as she saw Lee.

'Oh Dr Forrester, how nice to see you. Do come in and see if you can talk some sense into Dr Jameson. I'm sure I've done my best and all I get for my pains is a reminder to keep my place.' She clucked unhappily. 'Did you ever hear anything like it? Me, to keep my place. Well I'm sure I've known it these past fourteen years and I don't need to be taught it now.'

Lee felt her spirits sink. 'Why, whatever is wrong?' She hurried in, quickly depositing gloves and bag on the hall table. 'I'm sure he doesn't mean to snap at you, Mrs Dawson. It's not like him.'

'Bless you, I know that, and that's why I don't like it. I know he's not himself when he gets like this, but the more I try to tell him the worse he gets. Just like a child he is and him as ought to know better.'

Trying to hide a feeling of alarm Lee smiled. 'Doctors are always notoriously bad patients.'

'That's just it, he refuses to accept that he's a patient at all. I caught him just now on top of a step ladder taking all the books off the shelves in his study.'

'Oh no.'

'Oh yes. Coming down the steps he was, arms piled high and wobbling all over the place. I couldn't bear to look.' Mrs Dawson flapped her hand as if flapping the vision away. 'And he's puffing like an old grampus. Perhaps you can talk some sense into him, Doctor, because I'm sure I can't, and I don't intend to get my head bitten off for my pains. I'll go and make some tea. At least I know where I am in my kitchen.'

She stormed off huffily, leaving Lee to find her own way into the study with a lecture already framing on her lips. It faded abruptly as she saw

Tom sitting in the large leather chair, his eyes closed, his breathing deep. For a moment her heart pounded as she went quietly towards him but his eyes flickered open as she stood uncertainly. For a moment he appeared confused, then he blinked in recognition and snapped, crossly, 'I hope that interfering old woman hasn't sent you to give me a lecture, because if she has you can save your breath and I'll give her a piece of my mind.' He broke off, wheezing, and Lee tried to keep from her expression the sudden and very real concern she felt as she moved to sit calmly in the chair opposite.

'Not at all,' she said, smoothly. 'Why on earth should you think that, unless of course you've been doing something which you think deserves a lecture?' She pointedly eyed the piles of books and heard him grunt.

'Damn lot of fuss about nothing. A man can't even do as he pleases in his own house without some woman chasing after him.'

'If you mean Mrs Dawson, aren't you being a little unfair,' she prompted gently. 'As for interfering, she worries about you and you know you aren't supposed to be over-exerting yourself.'

'Rubbish. A little exercise is good for me.'

'Yes, within reason, I agree, but I'm sure the doctors didn't quite have in mind that you should climb ladders carrying arms full of books, or are you trying to add a broken leg to your list of achievements?' She eyed him firmly and he had the grace to look sheepish.

'So you have come to lecture me?'

'Not at all. As a matter of fact I came to see how you are. Father was asking.'

'Asking you to keep an eye on me?'

'You know better than that, and so does he, but that doesn't mean he isn't interested.'

'Well you can tell him I'm fine, never better.'

Lee fixed him with a meaningful stare. 'I'd like very much to be able to do that, and I will, if you'll promise me you'll just stop climbing ladders and behave sensibly.' She frowned. 'What were you trying to do anyway?'

'What does it look like?'

'Frankly, as if you were intending to rearrange the room.'

'Not the room, just the books. Why is it that the ones I want are always out of reach? I've been meaning to do it for years. The ridiculous thing is, then it didn't matter. Now it does.'

She looked up with relief as Mrs Dawson came in with a tray and a look passed between the two of them.

'And you needn't look like that.' The old man helped himself huffily to a cup and the only chocolate biscuit on the plate. 'You needn't think for one minute that I'm fooled by your little conspiracy.'

'I don't know what you're talking about Uncle Tom, there isn't any such thing and you know it. We just don't like to see you taking unnecessary risks, that's all. In any case if you asked him I'm sure Grant would be only too pleased to move the books for you.'

'He's got his hands full enough as it is. How are you two getting on, by the way?'

She stirred sugar noisily into her cup. 'Fine. It's working out very well.'

'Yes, he said it was.'

A crumb caught in her throat and she spent the next few minutes coughing, but at least it diverted his thoughts to other things. Before she left she spent half an hour re-stacking books onto different shelves. The job was almost complete when she heard a car in the drive and minutes later Grant walked into the room. He didn't seem particularly surprised to see her but he had probably seen her car parked outside. With barely a glance in her direction he examined the tea pot and poured himself a cup before proffering the pot in her direction. She shook her head.

'No thanks, I've already stayed longer than I intended. I must get back.'

'Ah yes.' He leaned nonchalantly against the door. 'I forgot, you have a date, well I'm sure you won't want to keep Charles waiting.'

Her lips formed a hard, teeth-baring smile as she brushed a hand across her face, conscious of the dust which had settled on her from the books.

'That's right, Doctor, I won't.' She walked to the door. 'By the way, give my regards to Miss Latimer.' She didn't wait to see what effect her parting shot had. The growl in his throat was sufficient to send her almost running out to the car, then she laughed involuntarily as she started the engine. 'One to me I think, Dr Sinclair.' Though for some reason there was little satisfaction to be found in the thought.

Charles gazed with undisguised admiration as she performed a twirl for his benefit. 'I hope this meets with your approval, sir?'

'I'll say it does.' Taking her in his arms he kissed her and she returned the gesture passively. She wasn't going to allow the evening to be ruined by Grant Sinclair. All the same, she couldn't help wondering how he would have reacted had she gone to so much trouble for his benefit instead of Charles', and then came an uncomfortable awareness that, in a way, it almost had been for his benefit. A kind of defiant gesture, which would serve no useful purpose at all she reminded herself crossly, because he wouldn't be there to see it.

She was unaware that she sighed involuntarily until Charles held her at arms' length and studied her with anxious eyes. 'What's the matter? You do want to go tonight, don't you? I did rather push you into it.'

She laughed awkwardly, cross with herself for having let her thoughts show. 'Yes, of course I want to go. I'm just not very good with crowds of people I don't know. I find it a bit daunting.'

'Oh, is that all? Well you don't need to worry. It's

not exactly a crowd. Just six of us. Jim Mortimer, he's with the local farmers' union, and his wife Anne. It's their party and you'll like them. And there's Steve Andrews and his fiancée. Steve works for the surveyors' department so I see quite a lot of him and Kathy's a librarian so if you need any reading material any time I'm sure she'll be able to help.'

'Don't talk to me about books,' she groaned and related sparingly the details of her afternoon while he finished his drink and she hunted for her evening purse.

It was a relief to discover that the Mortimers were indeed nice, ordinary people who went out of their way to make their guests feel at home and welcomed Lee like an old friend. Anne Mortimer led her upstairs 'to freshen up while the men pour out some drinks', and she sat on the bed chatting as Lee flicked a comb through her hair and checked her make-up.

'I'm so glad you could come,' she said. 'I know doctors are notoriously busy people.'

'I imagine farmers must be too. Charles tells me your husband is a member of the local farmers' union.'

'Yes, he is. Chairman actually,' she boasted with a pride which lit up her attractive face. 'It takes up a lot of his time but he enjoys it and so do I really. It's nice to know what's happening in your own area and generally to be aware of the things that may affect not only yourself but your neighbours' lives.'

'It sounds like a very responsible job.'

'Oh it is, only take my advice, don't get Jim started on the subject or he'll talk all night and I've told him once if I've told him a thousand times, mucking out the cows and dipping sheep don't make for ideal dinner table conversation.'

Lee laughed. 'There are times when I have pretty much the same problem with my own job.'

'Well, we'll do our best to steer clear of forbidden topics between us, shall we?' She watched as Lee smoothed her dress and looked woefully at her own more ample figure. 'I'm afraid being a farmers' wife leads me into all kinds of temptation. Jim needs a good hot cooked breakfast and another big meal later in the day. So do the farm hands when they've been out in all weathers, so I'm constantly cooking and eating. I keep promising myself I'll diet but somehow the right moment never seems to arrive.'

'I wouldn't worry. You look fine and obviously healthy and, what's more important, I'm sure Jim likes you just the way you are.'

'That's exactly what I tell myself,' Anne chuckled. 'I see we're going to be firm allies. Come on, let's go and see whether they've got round to the Common Market yet.'

They went downstairs just as the doorbell rang and Steve Andrews arrived with his fiancée. She was a pretty girl to whom Lee took an instant liking and even found herself promising to become a temporary member of the local library. 'Even though I'm not really sure how long I shall be in the area.'

She wondered whether she had imagined the quick glance which passed between Kathy and Charles.

'Yes, Charles tells me you've taken over from Dr Jameson until he gets over his heart attack.'

'Yes, that's right.'

'It was a tremendous shock to the people round here. Most of them have known him all their lives. He *is* going to get better?'

Lee sipped at her drink, trying to banish from her mind the picture of him as he had been that afternoon. 'I hope so. He'll need to be careful of course.'

'And you'll be staying in Foxley until he's well enough to work in the practice again. I know that Charles, for one, is delighted.'

Lee stumbled over an answer, partly because she didn't want to become involved in any professional discussion and partly out of confusion as she saw Charles glance in her direction with the kind of look which seemed to be asking her something she was not prepared to answer, at least not yet. She smiled. He was looking particularly nice in a dark suit and the lights picked out the few strands of grey in his hair, making him look rather distinguished. It was the first time she had really been consciously aware of the age difference between them, not that that sort of thing meant much these days and there was even something quite comforting about the way he rested a gently proprietorial hand on her arm.

'I've made no secret of the fact that I'd very much like you to stay,' he said, softly, as they followed the others into the sitting room for coffee after the meal, 'I hope you don't mind.' They stood chatting against a background of music coming from a subdued stereo.

'No, why should I?' But for some reason a vague feeling of embarrassment gave an edge to her voice and she looked up, suddenly serious. 'Please, Charles, don't . . . don't get too serious. Not yet, I'm not . . .'

'I know,' he cut her off quickly. 'It's too soon and I didn't mean this to happen, but I just want you to know that I've become very fond of you and I'd like to think there might be a chance that I could persuade you to stay.'

Lee felt her heart contract painfully, as if she were being dragged into something deeper than she was prepared to go at this stage.

As if aware of her thoughts he kissed her cheek. 'Look, it's nothing to worry about, especially now. I'm not asking you to marry me . . . not quite yet. The subject wouldn't even have come up if Kathy hadn't started dropping her rather heavy hints. But you know what small towns are. Everyone takes a hand in everyone else's affairs.'

Her mouth felt dry as she summoned a smile.

'More coffee anyone?'

Almost too quickly Lee held out her cup and

conversation became general again. She was very fond of Charles, she enjoyed being with him, but were they the kind of qualities which made for marriage?

She was even more relieved when they reached the cottage much later and Charles made no suggestion that he should come in. Instead he kissed her gently.

'It's been a lovely evening but I won't invite myself in for a night cap. I know you have to be up early, and so do I.'

Surrendering her mouth to his in a goodnight kiss, Lee felt a vague stirring of her emotions but they were emotions which defied analysis later as she lay in bed, staring into the darkness. She sat up, plumping the pillows crossly with her fist, and closed her eyes firmly. But not firmly enough to blot the image of Grant Sinclair out her thoughts completely. Blast the man! Why had he had to walk into her life, filling it with complications? He had no right, no right at all.

CHAPTER TEN

LEE woke next morning with a splitting headache and to the horrifying realisation that she had overslept. Maybe because she had had her mind on other things or simply because she had been tired, whatever the reason, she had somehow forgotten to set the alarm and consequently arrived at the surgery breathless and having had no breakfast as well as being ten minutes late.

Any hopes that she might have had of being able to get in quietly were dashed as Grant appeared just as she was making her apologies to Margaret. For an instant their eyes met and she knew he was angry. The fact that, in this instance, his anger certainly was justified made it if anything worse and she scuttled to her room, glad that he was too busy tracing a patient's cards at that moment, thus giving her at least a temporary respite.

Somehow she managed to get through the morning's list. Most of the patient seemed to be suffering from 'flu with all its varying symptoms and she found herself wondering why they didn't simply take to their beds using whatever kind of remedy suited them best rather than coming in to the surgery. Her own headache had reached thudding proportions and as she went gratefully in search of coffee later, she took her own advice and was just swallowing two aspirins when Grant walked in.

Looking at him she experienced a brief sense of shock. He looked as if he had scarcely slept, which, she told herself resignedly, might account in part at least for the note of biting irritability in his voice, but she certainly wasn't prepared for the bitterness of the attack he launched upon her.

'I take it you had a good evening, but forgive me if I express the hope that you don't intend making a habit of bringing your hangovers to this surgery, Doctor. It hardly provides a suitable image for the patient any more than arriving late does, and frankly, if you can't keep your working commitments and your social life apart, then you're not doing your job properly and you're no use to me.'

For a moment she was too stunned and angry to speak. His gaze was searing as he looked at her, no doubt taking in the shadows beneath her eyes, but if he thought she was going to accept meekly being judged and convicted without saying a word in her own defence then he had another think coming.

'Now just a minute.'

'No, I don't think so, Doctor.' His eyes snapped angrily. 'We seem to have wasted enough time already this morning. I've got calls to make. I imagine you have too, and in any case I'm not interested in excuses.'

She stood facing him, breathing hard. 'Which is just as well, because I'm not offering any.' She saw the momentary narrowing of his eyes and ignored it. 'I overslept because I forgot to set my alarm. Admittedly it was stupid of me . . .'

'Well at least you admit that.' His voice sneered and she had to resist a strong urge to slap his arrogant face, then found herself wondering if her thought had actually precipitated the action as he pressed a hand to his head and swayed slightly.

Concern briefly overcame other instincts as she watched him. 'Are you all right? You look awful.' It was true. His face was ashen, but she was in no mood to offer sympathy after the things he had just said.

'Yes, of course I'm all right,' he said, peevishly. 'It's just this damned headache.'

'A hangover perhaps?' she suggested caustically, and, taking the bottle of aspirin from her bag, slapped it firmly into his hand. 'I can recommend a couple of these. They do marvellous things for sore heads. I suggest you take several, Doctor, and now, if you'll excuse me, I have work to do.' She turned briskly on her heel, vaguely aware that he called after her, but she continued to walk away.

'So much for a truce,' she muttered as she slipped the car into gear and drove away. 'Next time I'll wave a white flag but knowing Grant Sinclair he'll probably shoot first.' A decision which did nothing to lift the cloud of depression which seemed to hang over her for the rest of the day.

Even the cottage didn't seem to offer the usual welcome when she returned to it. Probably because it was Mrs Slater's day off which meant that the fire wasn't lit and the debris from the various cups of coffee still littered the kitchen.

Sighing, she abandoned her coat, put a match to the fire which at least soon flickered into life, switched the kettle on and rushed upstairs to change into a comfortable pair of jeans and a sweater. Her reflection stared back at her, ridiculously child-like. Unfortunately, she decided crossly, there was nothing she could do about that and she tied a scarf over her hair before going downstairs to begin a vigorous but totally unnecessary assault upon the furniture with polish and duster.

It was late afternoon before she finally perched on a kitchen stool to eat a hasty meal of beans on toast. Eyeing the plate with a distinct lack of enthusiasm she forced the food down and was just carrying the plate to the sink when the door bell rang.

Frowning, she dried her hands on the frilly apron she was wearing. 'Now who on earth can that be?' Her glance went to the clock. It was probably Charles. No one else knew she was here, but the smile she was wearing vanished instantly as she opened the door and stared instead into Grant Sinclair's face.

He returned her stare, a flicker of amusement briefly twisting his mouth, and her hand flew involuntarily to the scarf covering her hair, dragging if off roughly, leaving her curls flattened and dishevelled. She guessed she probably had a smut on her nose too because he was looking at her with the kind of critical appraisal which left her blushing and wishing she had at least had time to put on a smear of lipstick. But it was just typical of the man to arrive unannounced.

She purposely made no attempt to invite him in, even when he glanced up at the sky and stood with the rain pouring over his face. It gave her some kind of satisfaction to see him shiver and turn up the collar of his coat. He looked like a bedraggled puppy, she thought, and it serves him right too.

He was clutching a package. A plant, judging from the sodden paper which was gradually disintegrating in his hands. A present for Miss Latimer. Poison ivy, no doubt. The thought flickered ungenerously through her mind as she said briskly, 'Forgive me if I don't invite you in but I'm rather busy, so if this is a social call . . . I'm still trying to get settled in.'

He peered over her shoulder to where the fire blazed and a vague spasm of guilt ran through her only to be crushed quickly. 'Yes, so I see.' Rain dripped from his hair. 'It looks very cosy . . . and warm.'

'Yes, it is.' Her smile was frosty. 'Except when the door is wide open. Now, is there really something I can do for you, Doctor, or is this simply a continuation of this morning's discussion because if so, to quote your own words, I object to mixing my business and social life?' The door was half closed when his hand shot out preventing her from shutting it completely. She rounded on him furiously. 'Now, look here . . .'

The plant wavered beneath her nose. 'This is for you.'

She stared at it, and at him. He looked awful. His eyes were sunk into their sockets and his features were taut with cold. 'For me? Is this some kind of joke?'

He held the collar of his coat tightly against his throat and she noticed that his hands were shaking. 'No joke. I'm afraid it's the best I could think of by way of an apology, and I really do apologise for the things I said this morning. I can only offer the excuse that I was feeling lousy . . . and still am for that matter.'

'Frankly, you look it.' He was leaning against the door, his eyes closed, and she had to dart out a hand to steady him as he swayed. To her consternation she could feel the heat of his body burning even through his sodden clothes. 'For heaven's sake, you're burning with fever.'

He nodded, his weight resting almost fully upon her now as in desperation she flung the plant onto a table beside the door and struggled to help him inside. Her foot pushed the door to a close, sending a waft of smoke billowing from the fire. 'Why on earth didn't you say something? You're ill.'

He smiled weakly and she was alarmed to feel him shaking violently. 'I always . . . seem . . . to say the wrong thing.' He closed his eyes again and she saw the beads of sweat on his face where he had brushed the rain away. 'God, I feel awful.'

'Here, lean on me.' She gasped as he took her at

her word and somehow managed to manoeuvre him towards the sofa where he collapsed, lying back with a hand flung over his eyes. She thought for one awful moment that he had passed out until he spoke.

'Sorry. I can't think what . . .'

'For heaven's sake, just don't talk. Let me help you off with your coat and shoes.'

He protested as she knelt and tried to ease off his shoe. 'Got to go.'

Grimly she eased him out of his coat. 'Somehow I don't think you'll be going anywhere. In fact, I rather think you have a very bad dose of 'flu.' He was a dead weight as she struggled to release his arm from the coat but finally she managed it and reproached herself as she carried it, dripping, into the kitchen and hung it over a chair. 'And you'll probably get pneumonia as well, thanks to me.' Fury with herself turned to consternation as she returned to the sitting room to find him lying full length on the settee, his shirt tugged open at the neck, his hair, darkened by rain, flattened against his head. Without thinking she bent to brush it back and almost gasped as some powerful emotion surged through her, like an electric current.

Biting her lip she backed away and looked at the recumbent figure, crossly. 'This is all very well, Doctor, but just what am I supposed to do with you? You certainly can't stay here.'

He didn't answer. She hadn't expected him to. He was out cold, snoring gently, and from the looks of him would probably stay that way for hours.

'Damn.' She flopped into the chair opposite and sat watching the sleeping figure. The thought came to her that it was odd that she hadn't been able to imagine Charles in the cottage completing a picture of domestic bliss, and yet now, for some ridiculously inexplicable reason, a curious feeling of well-being began to steal through her, as if the missing piece of a jigsaw had slipped into place. She studied him. He looked younger when he was asleep, more vulnerable somehow, as if Grant Sinclair could ever be vulnerable. She saw the faint lines around his eyes and wondered what had put them there. A woman perhaps? Miss Latimer?

The picture faded and she got to her feet, going into the kitchen to fill a hot-water bottle. There was only one thing wrong with this jigsaw puzzle. Someone kept coming along and smashing it to pieces and just when she thought she had rebuilt it again, it was only to discover that the most important piece of all was missing completely. But that was always the way with jigsaws.

Her hands shook as she draped a blanket over him, tucking the hot water bottle in beside him. As she did so he turned over, groaning in his sleep, and without warning his hands gripped her, drawing her close. She gasped and fell heavily against the sofa and his grip tightened as he muttered, 'Don't go . . . nice and warm. Stay here.'

She gritted her teeth, struggling with a protest but was silenced as his mouth closed commandingly over hers. She felt the warm, muscular strength of him as he held her closer. He was strong and the more she fought the more demanding his mouth became and with a sob she became still, feeling the passion build in him as if fed by some kind of desperation and gradually her own responses changed. Her mouth answered the hunger in his. For a moment almost as if he sensed it he became taut, then with a groan he drew her closer still until she felt she would be suffocated and had to force herself gently out of his grip to sit, breathing hard, on the floor beside him. He was delirious of course, didn't know what he was doing. With a sob she lowered her face into her hands and let the tears pour down her cheeks. For some reason she felt cheated. In the morning he wouldn't remember a thing about what had happened. Which was probably just as well. The thought brought a faint blush to her cheeks as she turned to look at him. He was sleeping deeply. His grip on her hand relaxed and she felt the tautness slip from his face. After a while she released herself gently and went upstairs to change into her nightdress and a warm dressing gown. It was going to be a long night. The first and last she would spend with Grant Sinclair and he wouldn't remember a thing about it.

It was about three in the morning when she woke and lay for a moment trying to remember where she was and why. Her arm had gone to sleep where she had fallen asleep with it pressed against the arm of the chair under her cheek. But it wasn't that which had woken her.

It was only as she shivered that she realised the fire had almost gone out and her gaze flew to the sofa where Grant lay. The blanket had slipped to the floor and he was moaning restlessly with cold. With a gasp of alarm she got to her feet and regretted the hasty movement as the circulation began to flow sluggishly in her limbs. She put a hand on his forehead and was shocked to find him icy cold. Quickly she knelt before the fire, stirring the ashes with a log, found a spark and put the wood into it, blowing gently to coax a flame. It started to crackle and the pale, flickering light threw shadows onto Grant's face. If anything she thought he looked worse, though it might have had something to do with the fact that he needed a shave. She found herself staring at the faint stubble on his chin and wondering what it was about men that made them look so helpless when they were ill. He lay with a hand thrown restlessly against the cushion she had put beneath his head, and the dark hair fell forward over his face which seemed so different now that all trace of cynicism had been swept from it.

Smiling to herself it was some seconds before she realised that his eyes were open and that he was actually staring up at her. Startled she became aware of what an incongruous figure she must look in the old, woolly dressing gown which she had flung on over her nightie, rather than spend the night fully dressed. Her eyes felt heavy from a lack of proper sleep and for a moment she panicked. How on earth was she going to cope with surgery in the morning? Obviously she couldn't leave him here alone. Perhaps Mrs Slater would come in. 'And how do I explain you to her,' she murmured, biting at her lip, then remembered with a sigh of relief that tomorrow . . . today, was Saturday.

'Cold.'

She felt herself jerked from the half drugged stupor as he spoke and hurried into the kitchen to make warm milk and carry it with two aspirin back to the sitting room where she found him tugging at the blankets. Disentangling him, she helped him to sip at the milk, supporting him gently. 'Here, take these with it, they'll help bring your temperature down.'

He managed it, with an effort, and she knew by the heat of his body that he still had a temperature despite the fact that he was shivering violently.

He lay back. 'Sorry about this. Can't think what happened.'

She surveyed him as if he were a schoolboy. 'Well, I'd say that you have a pretty hefty dose of 'flu, probably made far worse by the fact that you must have been struggling against it for days. Why on earth didn't you say anything?'

He closed his eyes. 'Didn't want to give in. Thought it might go away.'

She snorted with disgust. 'And I thought you

were supposed to be a doctor. Is that the kind of advice you give to your patients?'

He looked at her. 'You're a bully, you know that?'

Her mouth compressed. 'It's time someone took you in hand.'

'Are you volunteering for the job? If so I accept.'

She blushed furiously even as she told herself that it was all just the fever talking. A belief confirmed as he started to shiver again and tugged restlessly at the blankets.

'I'll be going soon,' he muttered. 'Just so damned cold. Can't seem to get warm.'

Lee prized the blanket from his grasp, doing her best to tuck it round him so that he couldn't throw it off again, but it was useless. He was still surprisingly strong so that just when she thought she had managed to tuck him in securely, he turned and she found the blanket in a heap on the floor again.

Sighing with exasperation and tiredness she gathered it up and tried again. 'Look, this is for your own good. If you think I'm going to see you catch pneumonia and end up here as a permanent guest, you've got another think coming. Life is quite complicated enough thank you very much.' She straightened up, eased her back and tried again, then gasped as the breath was knocked out of her as his hand shot out. She fell, swearing softly under her breath.

'You're making this very difficult, Doctor.'

His teeth were chattering. 'Cold.'

In exasperation she scrambled to her knees again, clutching the blanket. She leaned forward to tuck it over his shoulders and suddenly found herself grasped in a bear-like hug. With a loud screech she tried to detach herself, feeling his unshaven chin rasp her face, then he sighed and relaxed, clutching her as if she were a doll.

'That's nice. Warm.'

She gritted her teeth, tears of tiredness and a mixture of pent-up emotions flooding through her as she stared at him until it occurred to her that she was fighting a losing battle. 'Oh well, if that's what it takes to get both of us a good night's sleep . . .' She eased herself onto the sofa beside him. It was uncomfortable and she lay perched on the edge, stretching her legs out, scarcely daring to breathe. 'I must be mad,' she muttered into the darkness, but his breathing had steadied and gradually his shivering stopped.

She had just closed her eyes telling herself she would just doze when his arm shot round her and she squeaked as she felt herself dragged towards him. With fire burning in her cheeks she felt her body moulded against his own, trapping her so that she couldn't move. Slowly his hands explored the soft roundness of her body beneath the thin nightie she was wearing and she gasped with indignation, then he muttered something and lay still. Beneath the arm he had flung about her waist she lay staring into the darkness breathing hard and feeling the tears prick at her lashes until finally she remonstrated with herself aloud. 'Oh for heaven's sake go to sleep. Even if you get ravished in your virgin bed, he's not going to remember a thing about it.' She gulped and felt a tear slide down her cheek, not knowing whether it was anger or regret that put it there.

CHAPTER ELEVEN

HE WAS still sleeping when she crept into the kitchen the following morning. Glancing at him she saw the tousled head and felt her throat tighten. He looked like a young boy now that the fever had finally gone and he had relaxed.

She left him snoring gently, and began to break eggs into a bowl, switched on the coffee and popped bread into the electric toaster. Minutes later she heard his sharp exclamation and going to the doorway saw him sitting up surveying the sofa, herself and his surroundings with total bewilderment. There was something almost laughable about the way he sat with the blanket tucked over his knees.

He rubbed at his eyes and the growth of stubble on his chin as she emerged from the kitchen carrying a mug of coffee which she handed to him. 'How the hell did I get here? What's going on?'

'Don't you remember? You've been ill. As for why here,' she nodded in the direction of the couch, 'you turned up on my doorstep clutching a plant as a peace offering and promptly collapsed. Short of sending for an ambulance and having you carted off to the local hospital, which seemed rather drastic, there didn't seem to be much else I could do with you, so you slept here. On the couch.'

He stared at her incredulously. 'You mean all night?'

'Every hour of it.'

He groaned, took a long gulp of coffee as if it might clear his senses and looked at her again. 'Look, I'm sorry, I must have caused you a hell of a lot of trouble.'

'More than a little,' she was tempted to say as she rushed into the kitchen to rescue the toast and called to him through the open door, 'I coped.'

There was silence for a moment and when she returned he was sitting on the edge of the sofa, head in hands, but at least he had his feet on the floor, even if it did look as if he regretted the action.

'I'd take it easy for a while if I were you,' she prompted. 'Don't do anything too hasty too soon.'

He groaned. 'Frankly I don't think I'm capable of it. I feel as weak as a kitten.'

Remembering his strength last night she chose not to answer. 'Could you manage something to eat? Some toast or something a little more substantial?'

The question went unanswered as he stared with dawning horror at his clothes, or rather lack of them, and a scandalised expression filled his eyes. 'What the . . . who the devil removed my clothes?'

She couldn't help the laughter which tugged at her lips. 'Oh come on. I am a doctor you know. I've seen a man's body before now. In any case I simply removed your trousers and shirt because you were running a high temperature. I assure you, you're perfectly decent.'

With a strangled howl of indignation he dragged the blanket angrily around him and she choked back the laughter. 'Well I don't feel decent. I need a bath and a shave and as soon as I can make it I'll get out of your way.'

She bit her lip. He needn't have said it quite so eagerly. 'The bathroom's upstairs. Help yourself. Oh and you'll find your clothes on a hanger in the bedroom.' She turned away as he moved unsteadily to the door. He paused.

'Look, I am grateful. I realise . . . well I realise this is . . .' He broke off. 'Look I'm trying to say I'm sorry and thanks.'

'There's no need.' She kept the response purposely light, almost flippant and was glad to be able to give her attention to buttering the toast while he went upstairs to dress. She swallowed hard. It was ridiculous but suddenly she hated the thought of the emptiness after he had gone. Standing at the cooker preparing breakfast for two seemed like the most natural thing in the world and she had a momentary vision of doing it for the rest of her life . . . Of lying in his arms . . .

The memories came rushing back and she jumped violently as he was suddenly behind her, his hand on her shoulder.

'You have every right to be angry.'

'I'm not angry. Why should you imagine I would be?'

His eyes searched her face far too intently for comfort. 'Well, we haven't exactly hit it off have we, and then suddenly you find yourself landed with me as an unannounced, unwelcome visitor, spending the night on the couch . . .' He frowned and she looked away from the question she saw beginning to form in his mind.

'You weren't any trouble.' She rushed in to forestall it. 'You slept most of the time.'

His grip tightened fractionally on her arm as she tried to ease herself away. He glanced round the room and she bit her lip as she followed his gaze to the chair where the cushions were still piled up as she had left them and she cursed herself for not having tidied them before he woke. She saw the thoughtful expression edge its way into his eyes as if he was trying to remember.

'And just how much sleep did you get last night?'

'I managed perfectly well. I dozed.'

'In the chair?' Suddenly there was a hint of laughter in his eyes. 'That can't have been very comfortable.'

'It's a large chair.' Why did she sound so breathless? His eyebrows rose.

'So it is, and you're not exactly large are you?' Furiously, she knew he was laughing at her and before she could anticipate his intention he had pulled her towards him and the choking sound in her throat died as his mouth closed over hers. For an instant she tried to protest, but her parted lips merely seemed to invite his invasion of her mouth and senses. His grip tightened, imprisoning her, and she gasped as her body reacted to the sheer maleness of him, just as it had before. Against her will she felt herself respond. There seemed no point in denying that she loved him, any more than she could deny to herself that if he had tried to make love to her last night she would have let him.

With a gasp of horror she realised what she was doing. The fact that she wanted him wasn't enough, not when he was going to marry someone else. Shame made her stiffen in his arms and she felt almost faint with relief that he could remember nothing of what had happened, until he put her away from him, then she saw his expression change. She swallowed hard. Please God, don't let him remember.

'I'd better get the toast.'

But his hand still imprisoned her wrist. 'Don't run away from me, Lee. What are you afraid of?'

'Afraid?' Her laughter sounded shrill. 'Why on earth should you think that? Perhaps you're still a little delirious.'

'Was I delirious then?'

Why did she suddenly get the impression that he knew exactly what had happened? 'A little,' she said, frostily. 'But then, that's perfectly reasonable in someone with a high temperature.'

He was looking at her very oddly. 'I suppose you're right. I must have been. It's funny though, I distinctly recall feeling cold, very cold and then . . .'

Her voice came in a hoarse whisper, 'The mind can play all sorts of tricks. Patients often confuse things in their delirium with reality. You of all people should know that.'

'As you say,' he looked at her, coolly. 'It's hard to tell the difference but somehow I don't think I'm likely to make that kind of mistake, do you?'

Her answer was stifled as he kissed her. It was a protracted kiss which left her feeling breathless and shaken. The fact that he drew away, staring at her before releasing her gently, left her feeling irrationally depressed.

'I think it's time I left.'

She had to swallow hard so as not to cry. 'But what about your breakfast?'

His gaze swept her face. 'I don't think I'll bother, thanks. I've a lot of catching up to do.'

'Yes.' Her voice sounded brittle. With Miss Latimer no doubt. Suddenly she felt drained and tired. 'As a matter of fact so have I.' She looked round the room. 'Saturday is usually my day for catching up with the chores.'

'I'm afraid I upset your routine.'

He had upset far more than her routine, she thought. 'It doesn't matter.' A voice in her retaliated crossly. Yes it does. You barge your way into my life, turn it upside down and then walk out leaving me shaking like a jelly. She smiled weakly and he studied her, reflectively.

'I hope I didn't keep you from anything important.'

With a gasp of horror her hand flew to her mouth as she remembered she had promised to ring Charles. 'Oh lord . . .'

'I take it that means I did.' There was a sudden, definite coolness in his voice. 'It seems I owe you another apology, but I imagine you'll be able to put things right.'

Without giving her a chance to speak he was already gathering up his coat. 'I'll be going. Sorry about all the mess.'

She watched him walk out to his car and drive away before returning to the kitchen. The scrambled eggs had congealed in the pan. She stared at it and felt the tears prick at her eyes as she shovelled it furiously into the bin. 'Damn.' Her hand shook as she reached for the coffee pot, loading it with cup, milk and sugar onto a tray. Carrying it into the sitting room she sat on the couch. It was still warm and, instinctively, she pulled the blanket round her.

She drank two cups of coffee then grimaced and got to her feet. 'I don't even like coffee first thing in the morning.' Catching sight of her face in the mirror she stared at it with cold objectivity. There were shadows under her eyes and she was pale. 'I don't do a lot of things,' she told herself faintly, 'At least, I didn't.' The flush stole into her cheeks. She turned away and spent the rest of the morning trying to erase all trace of Grant Sinclair from her mind as well as from the cottage.

CHAPTER TWELVE

DRIVING to the surgery on Monday morning Lee found herself dreading the inevitable meeting with Grant. Not that he was likely to have remembered the events of the weekend any more clearly, she told herself, wishing it were possible to wipe them from her own mind so easily.

She felt tired, and worse, looked it. Charles had commented on it when he had come round for coffee last night and she had heard herself stumblingly telling him, without elaborating too much, what had happened. 'He just arrived and passed out. I had no choice but to let him stay.'

She had wanted sympathy and got it. That was the nice thing about Charles, she had found herself thinking as she relaxed against his chest as they sat on the couch. He was so uncomplicated, he could be counted on to stand firm, like a rock. Good old, solid Charles. Who wanted excitement anyway? She made an unsuccessful attempt to stifle her yawns and he got to his feet kissing her gently. 'Poor old thing. You should have told me and I wouldn't have suggested coming over for coffee.'

Guilt crashed like a huge wave. 'Oh no, that's all right. I'm just sorry I'm not better company.'

He looked at her with careful concern. 'Perhaps

you're going in for a dose of flu too. You look a bit rough.'

She had choked on an answer and said, yes, she would take a couple of aspirin and have an early night, and had done just that after he had left and she had cleared away the cups. But she hadn't slept, at least not until the early hours and then she had woken with the alarm, feeling cross and even more tired than ever.

And in the event she needn't have worried because Grant had only just arrived at the surgery too. He was just getting out of his own car as she turned the Mini into the drive. She sat, purposely foraging in her handbag, hoping he would go in ahead of her, but he turned back to collect some papers he had left on the back seat and as he straightened up, their eyes locked before he slammed the car door and strode away. He was still pale and she found herself wondering whether Christy Latimer was a good cook and if so why didn't she give him a good square meal, then reminded herself firmly that their domestic arrangements were none of her business.

He was standing holding the door open a little impatiently when she finally got out of her car. She noticed the envelope he was holding as she skipped through into the warmth and felt his arm brush against her sleeve. It was ridiculous the effect so slight a contact could have on her, yet his own expression didn't change by as much as the merest flicker of a smile. Which was in a way comforting because it confirmed that he hadn't remembered any more, but she was annoyed to find that her own cheeks were suddenly warm.

'Should you be back at work so soon?' Her voice was more brisk than she had intended and his brow rose. Surely that couldn't be laughter she saw in his eyes?

'What's this, concern for me? Why, I didn't know you cared.' He wasn't laughing, his eyes looked directly into hers and to her chagrin it was she who looked away.

'Of course I'm concerned,' she blustered, crossly. 'You were quite ill. I just thought you might need to spend a day in bed . . .' She floundered helplessly as his gaze fixed itself on her.

'I will admit the idea has its merits. Unfortunately I don't think it's justified. I'm fully recovered, thanks to your efforts. I was still a bit groggy yesterday. I don't know if I thanked you properly.'

She stared with agonised concentration at her watch and frowned. 'Yes, you did. Er . . . look I must go. I've phone calls to make before I see the first patient.'

'So have I.' His brow furrowed, then he handed her the envelope, almost as an after-thought. 'By the way, this is for you.'

She took it, recognising the handwriting as Tom's.

'It's an invitation to dinner. I've had one too.'

'You mean we're both . . .'

'We're both invited, yes, but not together if that's what's worrying you.' There was a sudden, caustic note in his voice. 'You're allowed to bring a guest. I shouldn't think that will present any problems.'

Any more than it would for him, she thought, and toyed briefly with the idea of refusing the invitation.

'Tom likes to have these informal get-togethers every now and again. I don't think we should disappoint him, especially now. Some kind of diversion is probably just what he needs.'

Again, his ability almost to read her thoughts put her immediately on the defensive. 'I wouldn't dream of disappointing him. I'll telephone him today and say I'll be delighted. Oh, but what about covering here if we're both off duty at the same time?'

'That's no problem. I'll get one of the local GPs to take any calls for the evening. It's a reciprocal arrangement. I've done my share and if there are any real emergencies we can always be reached.'

'That sounds fine.' But she walked away with the distinct feeling that she had somehow been manoeuvred. Still, it would be nice to see Uncle Tom again, even if she had to share the occasion with Grant and his girl friend.

She telephoned Charles who greeted the suggestion with enthusiasm. 'Yes, I'd love to come. I've a lot of time for old Tom Jameson. It will be nice to see him again and any excuse to spend an evening with you, darling, even if we won't be alone. I shall look forward to it.'

Lee smiled at the receiver. 'Yes, so shall I.'

'It just seems a bit hard that you have to spend an evening with Grant when you work with him all day. Poor darling. It's going to be a bit like coals to Newcastle for you, isn't it?'

'Oh well, I expect I shall be able to stand it. He's really not that bad, in small doses.' She heard Charles' laugh echoing her own.

'Till tomorrow night then.'

'Till tomorrow.'

She sighed and rang the bell for the first patient, wondering what Christy Latimer was likely to wear and mentally assessing the contents of her own wardrobe again. It was beginning to become a habit.

In the event she chose a dress in soft, cream-coloured angora wool. It moulded to her figure and a small scarf at her throat emphasised the colour of her hair and eyes. She had gone to endless pains shampooing her hair and applying a delicate touch of make-up to her face. The end results justified the effort if Charles' whistle of satisfaction was anything to go by as she came into the room carrying her bag and a small fur evening wrap.

Taking the wrap from her he draped it over her shoulders, his hands lingering as he brushed a kiss against her cheek. 'You look gorgeous. So gorgeous in fact that I don't know that I care to share you with anyone else. I'd much rather have you to myself.'

She turned in his arms, returning his kiss. The thought that he was going to be sitting beside her at Uncle Tom's gave her a comfortable feeling so that she relaxed. As if sensing a change in her Charles' kiss became more demanding. It was almost a silent moving of their relationship into a new phase. The knowledge left her feeling confused and she managed to evade him light-heartedly as he pulled her closer again. 'Hadn't we better go? We're due at Tom's in a quarter of an hour.'

He released her with obvious reluctance. 'I suppose you're right. I just wanted to be sure you know how I feel about you.'

'I think I do.'

'Oh damn, why on earth do we have to go out. There's so much I want to say.'

'We promised.' She laughed gently and fumbled in her bag for a comb. It was a relief to get into the car and to be able to sink back into the darkness where she could be alone with her thoughts if only for a little while.

Grant and Christy had arrived at the house before them. As she slipped off her wrap Lee heard their voices through the open door and caught a glimpse of Grant standing with a glass in his hand beside the girl who smiled up at him, looking staggeringly attractive in a dress which certainly hadn't been bought locally. With a pang Lee noticed how attractive Grant looked in the dark lounge suit. For a moment, as she stood in the hallway, his gaze rose and her heart thudded, then Tom was making them welcome, inviting them in and offering drinks.

'Everything's under control in the kitchen,' he reassured her. 'We've time for an aperitif, what will it be, my dear?'

'Sherry please. Dry.' She kissed his cheek. 'I think I'd better tidy up first.' She looked at Charles. 'You go in. I'll join you in a minute.'

She fled to the bathroom, her legs shaking, and leaned for a moment against the washbasin. This was ridiculous. There was a whole evening to get through and somehow she was going to have to smile and be polite, say all the right things, and pretend her heart wasn't breaking every time she looked across the table and saw Grant staring into the eyes of the woman he loved. It was crazy. Everything was getting out of hand. Somehow she had to pull herself together and get through the evening.

They were all talking animatedly when she returned to the lounge. Christy and Charles were engaged in a deep conversation and Tom excused himself on the pretext of seeing what progress was being made in the kitchen, leaving Grant to bring her glass of sherry. She took it, careful to avoid any physical contact, and sipped at it. His gaze followed hers.

'Tom looks well, doesn't he?'

'Yes he does.' In spite of herself she turned to

look at him. 'Were my thoughts really so obvious?'

'Only to me,' he said gravely, 'but then, I imagine we're both worried, both looking for the same thing.'

Her heart jerked uncomfortably. If only that were true. They moved towards the fire. Christy's gaze rose above Charles' shoulder and Lee noticed that her face briefly lost its animated look to be replaced by one of faint displeasure, but if he noticed there was no sign of it on Grant's face.

'Do you really think there has been an improvement?' She knew she was talking too quickly but at least this was safe ground.

'It's hard to tell. I've warned him that he has to be reasonable.'

'But does he listen?'

'You know him as well as I do.' His voice softened as he looked at her. 'You love him very much, don't you?'

'Yes, I do.' She couldn't prevent the slight quiver in her voice.

'Well, if it's any consolation, so do I. He's been like a father to me, so I do know what you're going through.'

She looked away, blinking hard. 'I don't think I could bear it if anything happened to him.'

'Then we mustn't let it, must we?' A large, firm hand closed over hers. She closed her eyes, then the glass was eased gently from her fingers. Her eyes flew open.

'You need to eat.' It was a statement rather than

a question. In fact, she hadn't eaten, but what right had he to know her so well? His mouth twitched and she relented.

'As it happens I'm starving.'

He laughed as Tom came back into the room and announced that they could eat. 'Well it looks as if we can do something about that at least.' His hand came down under her arm and her heart performed a crazy little dance. It faded into a dull bump as Charles came towards her and she found herself relinquished almost too quickly into his care, and for the rest of the evening she sat opposite Grant who seemed to direct the flow of conversation and easy laughter without noticing that she didn't manage to eat much after all.

They adjourned for coffee and Lee couldn't help noticing that he didn't seem to mind in the least the proprietorial manner in which Christy Latimer linked her arm through his, as if she was staking her claim. 'And why not,' she thought, dully, 'after all she has the right.' She turned her own attention on Charles, beaming at him, without having heard a word of what he had been saying for the past minute.

'Take it through into the library,' Tom directed. 'I'll be with you in a minute. I've a rather special bottle of brandy somewhere. Grant, help me look, there's a good chap. You know where I tend to leave it.'

They moved into the library, to find the room suffused by the glow from the fire and a solitary lamp. It was cosy, smelling of books and old leather. A tray of freshly made coffee had been left on one of the small tables. Lee moved towards it automatically, purposely avoiding looking at the clock, wondering how long it would be before she could reasonably make an excuse to leave. The meal had been lovely and cooked to perfection yet somehow it had all tasted like chaff in her mouth.

'Shall I be mother? Sugar, cream?'

'Leave it.' Charles drew her gruffly away from it and took her in his arms. She wasn't sure whether Christy had tactfully disappeared on purpose or whether she was helping Grant in his search for the brandy. 'It can wait for a few minutes, just while I kiss you and tell you how beautiful you are.'

He prised the coffee pot from her hands, putting it on the tray. He was really quite good-looking in a nice, gentle sort of way, she found herself thinking. Not like Grant's rugged looks of course, but then, not every woman went for the heavy, caveman type, she argued with herself crossly, allowing herself to be kissed. She felt a little light-headed. It was probably the wine. She had drunk more than she would normally have done because toying with the glass had provided cover for the fact that she wasn't eating, and now she felt almost comfortably detached from her earlier misery.

She felt a slight tug of shock at the apparent ease with which she abandoned herself to the effects of the wine, then decided she felt slightly sick and let her head rest against Charles' chest until the feeling passed, except that it didn't. Grant was right, blast him, she should have eaten a proper lunch.

She was jerked back to full awareness to find Charles manoeuvring her face up to his and kissing her soundly. It was a pleasant sensation, but it lacked the power to rouse her as Grant had been able to do. 'My God,' she thought, 'I'm assessing them as if they were bottles of wine.' She focused her gaze on Charles' tie and tried to concentrate on what he was saying.

'I love you, you know that. I've been trying to put it into words since the day we met. Well, the second time we met. On the first I was a little hazy but I knew even then that someone special had walked into my life.' He raised her face between his hands and kissed her again. The room was spinning and she felt oddly disappointed that it was the effects of the wine rather than the kiss. Perhaps if she closed her eyes and pretended it was Grant . . . Her mouth quivered hungrily. She felt Charles' momentary surprise before he responded, this time more fiercely, his mouth moving from her mouth to her ears, to her eyes.

'Darling, say you'll marry me.'

The bubble burst, she was only fooling herself that anyone could take Grant's place. She moaned softly, dimly aware as her eyes flew open of the figure standing in the doorway, the disbelief in his eyes turning to mockery and then open contempt as he took in her flushed cheeks and the glazed look in her eyes. She struggled to free herself from

Charles' embrace, feeling sick and conscious only of Grant's stony expression. It was all too obvious that he had drawn his own conclusions.

'Forgive me,' his voice was icy. 'I seem to have chosen the wrong moment to intrude.'

Her mouth opened to explain but it was too late, he was already turning on his heel and was gone before she could utter a word.

Sickness washed over her. He must have heard Charles' proposal but that could hardly account for the look of fury she had seen on his face. He knows I'm drunk, she thought, white-faced, as she pressed a hand to her head. But I'm not. You don't get drunk on two glasses of wine . . . and a sherry . . .

'I feel sick.'

Charles steered her quickly to a chair. She flopped into it and closed her eyes, gulping against the tide of nausea. 'I'm sorry, Charles, you were saying something . . .'

He smiled, wryly. 'Actually I was proposing, but I seem to have managed to get my timing all wrong, don't I.' He brushed the hair back from her face. She felt clammy and he was instantly all concern. 'Good lord, you're burning. I hope you've not got this wretched 'flu after all.'

'I shouldn't think so,' she said, weakly, too full of misery to care. She just wanted to go home to bed and have a good cry. 'It's the wine. It's gone to my head. I'm awfully sorry, Charles.'

'There's no need to apologise.' He straightened up. 'I still think you're not well. Anyway, I'm going to take you home. Will you be all right while I get your wrap?'

She nodded and the room moved again. 'I think so. I'm afraid Grant didn't look too pleased.'

'It's hardly our fault that he chose to walk in at the wrong moment.'

She tried miserably to convince herself that it hadn't been quite as bad as she imagined, and knew that it had. Her cheeks had been flushed, her eyes were too bright and he must have been sickeningly aware of the ecstasy in her eyes, but there was no way she could tell him that it had been him she was thinking of, not Charles.

'I don't suppose it was,' she agreed, numbly.

'In any case, Grant tends to have a bit of a chip on his shoulder where that sort of thing is concerned. A backlash, I suppose, from the girl he was engaged to.'

Lee felt her scalp tingle. 'Engaged?'

'Of course you probably don't know. Yes, he was engaged to a girl for about a year. They were planning to marry when they found out she had some incurable condition. I'm not exactly sure what it was but it was all very tragic. I don't think Grant has ever got over it properly.'

The room was spinning crazily as Lee sat up. She felt pity flood through her as she struggled to get to her feet, fighting the dull headache which had started to pound inside her skull. 'I didn't know.'

Charles' voice sounded miles away and she knew he was looking at her rather oddly. 'There's no reason why you should. He doesn't talk about it. Look, I think I'd better get you home. You look awful.'

She was happy to allow herself to be led into the hall and muffled in her fur wrap. Charles went in search of Tom, she heard the vague exchange of words, then they were being ushered out of the door into the cold night air with words of concern and reassurance ringing in their ears. From the car she looked back and held her breath. Grant was standing in the doorway. She couldn't see his features but could imagine the look of contempt in his eyes, then another figure came to stand beside him, smaller, slender. She reached up to say something, then, together, they turned and went back into the house, closing the door behind them as the car pulled away.

Lee was glad Charles made no attempt to come into the cottage. 'I think the best thing is for you to get straight to bed. Have a hot drink. I'll call you in the morning. Not too early.'

She managed a laugh. 'I should have slept it off by then.' Her lips brushed against his cheek. 'I really am sorry. I've made a fool of myself and spoiled your evening.'

'Nonsense, you haven't done either. I'm still not convinced it's the wine.'

She wasn't convinced either as she undressed and finally collapsed into bed. Suddenly she felt stone cold sober but her head ached and she swallowed two aspirin then switched out the light. She hadn't expected to sleep but her last thought was of Grant's face as he stood in the doorway with Christy Latimer beside him.

CHAPTER THIRTEEN

It took a real effort to drag herself out of bed next morning, but at least the dizziness had gone and some more aspirin brought the headache under control.

Surgery was mercifully light and she emerged feeling wrung out to drink a cup of coffee in splendid isolation, grateful that Grant had been called out and that she wouldn't have to face him yet awhile.

Margaret came through from Reception to find her staring lethargically out of the window. Snow had given way to fine sleet and it was blowing in whirling gusts against the trees. The thought of having to go out filled her with depression and she shivered. Perhaps Charles was right after all and she was going in for a chill.

'You look awful.'

Margaret's voice intruded and Lee drew herself up with a start. 'Sorry, I was miles away.'

'I said are you all right? You look terrible. Sure you're not going in for 'flu?'

'I shouldn't think so. Just a bit chilly, that's all, and a bit of a headache.' She shrugged herself into her cardigan, promising herself the luxury of a hot bath, a drink and an early night. 'It's probably a cold and a late night last night. I've taken some more aspirin.' Despite the fact that she seemed to have been swallowing them with daunting regularity for the past twenty-four hours her head felt remarkably whoozy and her glance went to the piece of paper Margaret was carrying with rueful anticipation. 'That's not a call for me, is it?'

''Fraid it is. Sorry.'

Lee sighed and read the details. 'Oh well, I don't think it's too urgent. I've several others. With a bit of luck I can fit it in on my way back.'

Margaret picked up the empty coffee cup, eyeing her pale face with some concern. 'You really don't look well enough to be taking surgery. Why not let me call Dr Sinclair, I'm sure he'd take over.'

'No.' Lee flinched at the sharpness of her own voice, then smiled. That last lot of aspirins didn't seem to be having much effect. 'Honestly, there's no need. He has a full work load as it is. Anyway, I'm off duty tonight so I'll pop back with these notes then go straight home to bed.'

'Well, if you're sure, but I don't think he's going to be very pleased.'

'Then perhaps we'd better not tell him,' she suggested, lightly, thinking that he was the last person in the world who should complain of her stubbornness after the way he drove himself into the ground.

She got into the car and headed for the first of her calls. She felt drained and knew that her eyes were dark ringed. By the time she was on her way to the second address it needed a real effort of will to go on, as if a steel hammer was pounding in her head, and her body shook in cold tremors. 'Come on now, pull yourself together,' she told herself sharply. She pulled up at the house and sat for a moment in the drive, gathering herself and waiting for a spell of dizziness to pass before getting out and walking on legs which felt like rubber to the door.

Ten minutes later, back in the car, she rested her head on her arms against the steering wheel for a minute before forcing herself to concentrate. One more call to go and that looked fairly routine. 'Just keep going,' she told herself as she headed along the narrow roads. 'Another hour and you can be home and in bed.'

She sighed and found herself relaxing her aching body at the mere thought. It was only when she felt the car thud against the grass verge that she realised, sick with horror, that she had actually almost lost consciousness. Heart thudding she fought to control the wheel and somehow managed to pull in at the nearest lay-by where she switched the engine off with hands which shook, then sat back, closing her eyes, letting everything spin crazily around her. It would pass in a few minutes. She passed a hand across her forehead and felt the burning. If only she had a drink of water or a flask of coffee.

She knew it was useless to try and go on. She felt herself slipping in and out of an uneasy sleep and every time she opened her eyes the car seemed to be spinning. Not knowing how long she had been sitting there she managed to drag her wrist up to her face and gasped. It wasn't possible. She must have been parked for a couple of hours without realising that it had actually begun to get quite dark. Her hand automatically fumbled for the lights, turning them on. The action allayed a feeling of panic but it was only temporary. She wasn't capable of driving, she would be a menace to herself and anyone else on the roads. But the thought of being stranded alone, in the dark, all night . . . She rested her head back against the seat, wishing Grant were there and the next thing she knew was that the door was being wrenched violently open and he was standing there his face ashen and angry as he lifted her from the seat.

Of course it was all part of the dream, she told herself, making no effort to resist as she felt herself bundled relentlessly into a blanket and carried. The fact that he didn't speak simply confirmed her belief. She felt too exhausted to ask herself why she could feel his heart pounding or why he looked so grim.

She protested just a little as he put her down and was vaguely aware that she was in his car, that he wore no jacket, just a sweater, and that the collar of his shirt was turned up, as if he had dressed in a hurry.

'Just sit still.' His voice brooked no argument as she began to protest. 'Have you any idea of the hell I've been through, wondering what had happened when you didn't get back to the surgery? Imagining all sorts of things.' She tried to argue that it wasn't her fault, but he gave her no chance. 'You little fool. Why didn't you say you weren't well? If Margaret hadn't told me . . .'

She stared at his grim face and burst into tears. It was too much, as if she didn't feel bad enough without having him bellowing at her like an angry bull.

With a muttered oath he had slipped his arm behind her and she felt herself held tightly. 'I'm sorry,' he brushed the tears from her face. 'I'm sorry, but if I hadn't found you . . . you might have frozen to death.'

If she hadn't been trapped in the warmth of the blanket she would have reached up to brush the hair from his face, to smooth the gaunt, anxious look from his eyes, but he held her against him. 'I'm afraid, my darling, that you've caught a nasty dose of 'flu and it's probably all my fault.'

It probably was, she thought, crossly, then anger faded as he kissed her, very gently. 'Don't worry, I'm going to take you home and see you tucked up safely in bed.'

'That will be nice,' she murmured contentedly, only protesting when the car slid to a halt and she found herself jerked out of a nice, comfortable position against his shoulder and a waft of cold air made her start to shiver again.

Mrs Slater's voice was full of concern, then Grant's intruded, briskly. 'I'll carry her upstairs if you'll make a nice hot drink and find a couple of aspirins. No, I can manage. We doctors are used to handling difficult patients.'

There was something about the way he said it. Difficult patient? She stared at him crossly. 'Please put me down. I'm quite capable of walking.'

He fixed her with a placid smile. 'If I put you down now, you wouldn't be capable of taking two steps under your own steam, so don't argue, there's a good girl. I know what I'm doing.'

The possibility that he might put her brave words to the test was suddenly too daunting to contemplate, but being in his arms was doing crazy things to her temperature and her head was spinning again.

Within minutes it seemed, someone was helping her to undress and slide between the blissfully cool sheets. The relief was exquisite. Suddenly she realised that her entire body was aching and she felt ridiculously close to tears again.

'I'm sorry,' she gulped. 'I'm sure I'll be all right in the morning.'

'Somehow I doubt that,' Grant said, quite calmly, and she opened her eyes to find him staring down at her with the kind of brooding expression which made her feel hot all over. She wondered when he had come up to her room, then there was a tap at the door and Mrs Slater came in with a mug of hot milk, clucking sympathetically as she put it on the bedside table and eyed Lee. 'You poor thing. It's horrible, this 'flu, but then I'm not surprised. You've been looking peaky for days.' Her glance rose to Grant. 'You managed all right then, Doctor?'

'Perfectly, thank you, Mrs Slater.'

Lee wondered briefly what he had managed, then gave up the attempt to work it out as his arm slid behind her and he held her while she finished the drink. Lying back she studied him sleepily. It was a pity about Christy Latimer, she thought. She wasn't his type at all. He needed someone who would look after him, cook him huge meals, darn his socks . . .

The phone rang. Mrs Slater's voice drifted up to her. She hoped it wasn't a call. She really didn't feel she could get out of bed quite just yet.

'Don't worry about it,' Grant's voice murmured soothingly in her ear, then she felt his lips brush against her cheek. She felt cheated. Her mouth had been ready for a kiss.

She shivered uncontrollably. 'I'm so . . . c . . . cold.' Her teeth chattered and she wondered why Grant's mouth suddenly became a taut line as he stood over her.

'Don't tempt me, my girl,' his voice rasped.

She frowned, then giggled. 'I promise I'll behave.'

There was no answering laughter. 'You don't know what you're saying, and even if you did, I'm not at all sure I could promise the same thing.'

Her eyes were bright as she looked up at him. 'I don't care.' She knew she was behaving abominably but somehow she didn't care. She heard his sharp intake of breath as he bent towards her, then Mrs Slater was in the room again, peering round the door, whispering.

'Oh Doctor, I'm sorry but there was a call . . . for Dr Forrester. It was Mr Mowbray. I explained that she's poorly and he said to give her his love and he'll call again tomorrow.'

Lee felt the happiness die within her as Grant's expression hardened. She began to cry quietly and for a moment her hand was enveloped in a stronger one.

'Don't go,' she sniffed.

There was a moment's hesitation before he answered and then his voice sounded strange. 'I think I'd better. You're delirious and I'm afraid if I stay I'll take advantage of the fact and you'd hate me in the morning.'

He rose to his feet, cool and withdrawn again. 'Remember me to Charles. Sleep tight, little one. I'm only sorry . . .'

She couldn't imagine what he was sorry about and suddenly felt far too tired to ponder on it.

CHAPTER FOURTEEN

'Hullo, Charles, yes I'm fine. Much better, thank you.'

'I was quite worried about you, darling. I was coming round but Mrs Slater said you were sleeping and Grant insisted you needed a real rest.'

'Grant did?'

'Yes, I spoke to him yesterday. He seems edgy but I suppose he's got his hands full with this epidemic.'

'Yes, I suppose that's it.' Her voice stuck in her throat. 'Still, I shall be taking my share again now, which should help. I feel so guilty, being ill now of all times.'

'My dear girl, you're far too conscientious. Why not take another day off?'

'But I've already had three.' She managed to laugh but it had seemed like three years, lying there, thinking, trying to get things into perspective. 'Charles . . . did you phone the cottage or did I imagine it? I know it sounds silly but things are so hazy.'

She could imagine him smiling. 'You didn't imagine it. I phoned to say thanks for a lovely evening at Tom Jameson's and Mrs Slater told me you were ill so I just said I'd call back.'

'I see.' She swallowed hard. So that part at least had been real, which meant that the rest . . . Her fingers toyed with the prescription pad. 'Charles . . .'

'Lee, I need to talk to you.' There was a sense of urgency about his voice which suddenly filled her with panic.

'I'm awfully busy right now, Charles. Will it wait until this evening or is it important?' She didn't know why she lied, except that for some reason she couldn't identify she didn't want him to say what she was sure he was going to say. There was a slight pause at the other end of the line and she hated herself for her cowardice.

'Actually it is rather important, unless you really would rather it waited.'

'No.' She closed her eyes. 'It's all right. I can make time.'

'It's just that, well, we were rather interrupted the other night and we never did exactly finish our conversation, did we?'

Poor Charles. She could hear the uncertainty in his voice and her hands tightened. 'No, I suppose we didn't.'

'I seem to be doing it again, getting my timing all wrong, don't I?' There was a hollow ring to his laughter. 'But I'd like to know . . . Lee, I do love you, you know that, don't you?'

'Yes, I think I do, Charles, but . . .'

'I know I'm rushing you.'

'Charles, I . . .'

'I know I'm not really being fair,' he was rushing on without giving her a chance to speak. 'But ever since we met I've been crazy about you and the other evening I was perfectly serious when I asked you to marry me.'

She felt as if the tightness in her throat would choke her. 'Yes, I realise that, Charles, and I'm very flattered, truly I am.' Why couldn't he realise that she was incapable of making a rational decision, any decision, right now. She caught sight of her face in the mirror, it looked thinner, drained.

'Lee, darling, I don't want to push but I'm going crazy, hoping you'll say yes. I know I could make you happy.'

'Dear, dear Charles.' She didn't doubt at all that if she married him she would be secure, cared for and loved. But was that enough?

'I'm sure you could.' Her voice sounded oddly flat. 'It isn't that . . . I'm very fond of you, very fond.'

There was a long pause and she felt like a murderess. 'You're saying "no", aren't you?'

'Oh, Charles, I wish it could be the way you want.' The words came out in a rush now. 'I have thought about it, and I do love you, in a way, but not that way.'

'Is it that I haven't given you enough time?'

'No, it isn't that.' She shook her head, hating the hurt in his voice.

'Is there someone else?'

She flinched, caught off guard. 'I . . . no, there's

no one else. As a matter of fact, I shall probably be leaving Foxley quite soon. You know my job was only temporary in the first place. Well I have to start looking for something more permanent. I've applied for a couple of posts.' It wasn't true but it was all she could think of to fill the silence and the irony of it was that she knew she would have to leave now anyway, because she couldn't bear to go on living and working close to Grant, knowing that his future was tied up in someone else.

Charles seemed to be waging some private war with himself at the other end of the phone. 'I hadn't realised Tom had made such a good recovery,' he said, leadenly.

'No, well he hasn't, not yet. But I agreed to take the job just for a few weeks on the understanding that both sides would be looking for an alternative. In any case Grant and I haven't exactly hit it off, you must have noticed.'

'I can't say I had. As a matter of fact I was almost beginning to get the idea that he had taken quite a fancy to you.'

'You must be joking.' In spite of herself she laughed. 'I think he has other plans and they certainly don't include me.'

'Well I can only say he's a fool.'

'Oh Charles . . .'

'No, don't say anything. I shall only start thinking you might change your mind, out of pity if nothing else.'

'You wouldn't want that.'

'It might be enough for me.' His voice rasped, then he said, with an attempt at lightness, 'Anyway, I'd better let you get back to your patients, their need is probably greater than mine, though I'm not entirely convinced of that at this moment.' There was silence then, 'Goodbye Lee, and good luck. We'll still be friends.' And the receiver clicked before she could say anything in reply.

Staring at it she had a momentary urge to call him back, to say she would settle for the terms he wanted, but it was no use. It was Grant she loved and there was no future at all in that, no future at all except to go away, try to pick up the pieces and start again.

With a little careful organisation she managed to avoid seeing Grant for the rest of the morning. Unfortunately as she returned later to collect some papers her heart missed a beat as she saw Christy Latimer's car parked in the drive. They had probably had a lunch date, the thought twisted like a knife as she hurried as quietly and quickly as possible through Reception and to her own room, cursing herself for having forgotten the papers.

The surgery was strangely quiet now that Margaret and the patients had gone. Chairs lined the waiting room in neat little rows, piles of magazines sat in tidy heaps, the carpet had been vacuumed. It all looked unnaturally clean and tidy and she had to battle against the sudden knowledge that she was going to miss it all. Worst of all she was going to miss Grant. There was going to be a huge void in her life which no amount of work could fill, but she had to try and the sooner she got away the better.

Lying awake last night she had reached the decision. It was simply a matter of choosing the moment to broach the subject. Tom would understand that she needed to look for something permanent. As for Grant, he would be only too pleased to see her go. She dropped the papers she had come to collect into her bag, snapping it to a close. It wasn't until she heard the muffled sound of voices as she crossed Reception that she realised Grant's door was open slightly. She heard Christy's voice quite clearly. It was shrill, tinged with annoyance.

'Darling Grant, you can't shut yourself away from the real world for ever. Beth is dead and you've got to get on with life. Yes, by all means treasure her memory, but you can't throw away any chance of happiness just because you're afraid it might happen all over again.'

Involuntarily Lee froze to the spot. She knew she should make her presence known, or just leave, but her feet wouldn't move, not even when she heard Grant's voice, suddenly very close, as if he was standing just at the other side of the door.

'You're right.' There was a ragged edge to the words. 'I suppose I've been kidding myself that I was honouring her memory in some way. I realise now that I was just being a coward.'

'Not a coward, a fool maybe.'

'I've always had the idea that I would be betraying her in some way by marrying.'

'Oh Grant, darling, don't you realise that that's exactly what Beth would have wanted, for you to start again, be happy?'

Lee drew in a deep breath, knowing she couldn't bear to listen to any more. Her hand was shaking as she reached the door. So it was settled then, he was going to marry Christy. Well in that case the sooner she got away the better, before she made a complete fool of herself.

To her horror the outer door creaked as she opened it. For an instant she froze, hoping it hadn't been heard, then suddenly Grant was standing framed in the doorway of his room, his face taut as he called after her.

'Lee, wait.'

She ran blindly, tears coursing down her face. She didn't want to hear what he had to say. He had every right to be angry that she had been eavesdropping, but what difference did it make how much she had heard. It wasn't as if he needed her blessing to marry the woman he loved.

She flung herself into the car, holding back the sobs, and drove off, tyres scraping the gravel. Casting a frenzied look in the mirror she saw to her relief that he had made no attempt to follow, which was just as well because her mouth felt too frozen to offer even a pretence at a smile of congratulations.

Later that evening after she had drawn the curtains in the cottage she sat down in front of the fire and tried to compose her letter of resignation. It was the hardest thing she had ever done and an hour later she was still unhappy with the results. But the brief, stiffly formal letter seemed the only way out. No excuses, no tears, or at least none that would be seen. A neat, clean ending.

She went to bed leaving the letter, ready stamped, propped against the clock and, in spite of her fears, fell asleep the moment her head touched the pillow.

She woke feeling slightly sick as the ringing of the telephone cut ruthlessly into a dream in which she was waiting for a train which never quite seemed to reach the station, and Grant was chasing her as she ran desperately to meet it.

Her hand brushed against the alarm clock. Catching it she stared at the hands. Three-fifteen! She jerked the receiver up, brushing a hand through her hair as she tried to gather her wits.

'Hullo, yes, Dr Forrester speaking.'

'Oh Doctor, thank heavens I've managed to reach you.' A woman's voice spoke coolly in her ear. 'This is Foxley General here. Sister Raymond speaking. I've afraid I've bad news.'

She was fully awake now, standing on legs that trembled. Not Grant, please God, don't let it be Grant.

'I'm afraid Dr Jameson has been admitted as an emergency, Doctor. He's had another heart attack.'

Lee felt her stomach tighten. 'He's not . . . ?'

'Oh no, Doctor.' The voice was calmly reassuring. 'But naturally with his past history we are very concerned, and Mrs Dawson, his housekeeper, felt you would want to be told.'

Lee sat weakly on the bed wishing her heart would stop pounding. She took a few deep breaths. 'Yes, I'm very grateful. Poor Mrs Dawson. Is she at the hospital now?'

'Yes, she is. We've made her comfortable and given her some tea but of course she's very upset. I gather she found the doctor. It was lucky she heard him and managed to get help so quickly, but I think she's probably in a fair state of shock herself and would be better off at home. I promised to get hold of Dr Sinclair to let him know. I've been trying for the past hour but he must still be out on a call so I rang you. I hope you don't mind, Doctor.'

'No, of course not. I'm glad you did. Look, I'll be over as quickly as possible. Please tell Mrs Dawson.'

'Yes I will, Doctor. I know she'll be pleased and perhaps you'll be able to persuade her to go home and get some rest.'

Lee rang off and began to dress without any thought as to what she put on. She found a pair of jeans and a shirt and sweater which she pulled on over the top. Her thoughts were in a turmoil. Tom had seemed so much better and now this. It was inconceivable that he should die and yet she knew enough not to fool herself that it wasn't going to be touch and go.

She drove to the hospital, praying that someone would have been able to contact Grant. It was going to hit him hard too and she wondered how she was going to face the look in his eyes, knowing that he had already been hurt so much, first losing the girl he had planned to marry and now this.

She drove into the car park where the lights cast a strange, fluorescent glow over everything. There was no sign of Grant's car, and her spirits sank. So they still hadn't been able to reach him. But if he was out with Christy they wouldn't, she thought, bleakly, then shut the idea out of her mind. It was none of her business what he did with his free time. But it was a lonely walk along the corridors, listening to the sound of her own shoes on the gleaming floors as she hurried towards the swing doors.

There was something touching, almost frightening about the way in which Mrs Dawson greeted her arrival. She looked older and had obviously been crying but her face broke into a smile of relief as she saw Lee and got to her feet.

'Oh Doctor, I'm so glad you've come. I didn't know what to do.'

'You did exactly the right thing.' Lee put her arm round the woman and led her back to the chair. 'Sister tells me you called the ambulance.'

'That's right. It was such a shock, finding him there like that. I heard him call out, you see, and when I went in there he was on the floor.' Her eyes filled with tears again. 'I knew Dr Sinclair was out and I didn't know what to do. He's going to be all right isn't he, Doctor? He looked so ill. I thought he was dead. He's not going to die is he?'

Lee bit her lip, not knowing what comfort she could give. Over the woman's shoulder she caught sight of a navy-blue clad figure coming towards them. 'I hope not, Mrs Dawson. I'm sure the hospital staff are doing everything they can and the fact that you got him here so quickly must help.' Her throat felt tight and painful. 'Here's Sister now. Perhaps they'll let me see Uncle Tom, then I might be able to tell you more, but in the meantime it really would be best if you went home and tried to get some sleep.'

Mrs Dawson clutched at her handbag. 'Yes, it's silly to wait isn't it, but I don't like to leave him somehow.'

'I know, but there really isn't anything any of us can do right now and you need to get some sleep. You're going to need all your strength once he starts getting over this.' She forced a laugh. 'You know what Uncle Tom is like.'

'I should, after all these years.' She gulped back a sob. 'Not that I shall sleep, mind, but you will call me if there's any . . .'

'I promise.' Lee's hand closed firmly on the woman's arm. 'As soon as I know anything or if there's any change.' Sister was catching her eye. There was still no sign of Grant and suddenly she wanted him there, very much.

She watched Mrs Dawson leave before turning to follow the neat navy-clad figure of the Sister.

'Tell me honestly, how is he? I'd like to know before I go in to see him.' She tried to smile but her lips felt stiff with tension. 'I promise I won't let him see that I'm upset.'

Sister Raymond considered her, gravely, slowing her steps a little. 'I'm sure you won't, Doctor. I'm afraid he's very ill. The attack was certainly more severe than the previous one.'

'Is he conscious?'

'He is, but I doubt if he will be able to talk to you and it's better if he doesn't try.' She paused outside the door. 'Doctor would prefer it if you don't stay too long.'

Lee's hand shook as she braced herself to enter the room. 'I won't. By the way, has anyone been able to contract Dr Sinclair yet?'

'Not yet I'm afraid, but we'll keep trying.' Sister smiled and nodded towards the door. 'Go in, Doctor. You'll find a chair by the bed if you want to sit with him for a few minutes. Nurse will be popping in every few minutes or so just to check on his progress.' She hurried away on soft-soled shoes and Lee walked slowly into the room.

She had imagined herself prepared but couldn't completely stifle a gasp of shock as she looked at Tom. He seemed somehow to have shrunk. Lying there, propped up against the pillows, he seemed to bear little resemblance to the man she knew, who had seemed so full of life only a few days ago. His face was grey and he lay with his eyes closed, taut with pain.

She sat in the chair, watching as he slept. A young nurse popped in and out of the room several times, smiled and went about her tasks soundlessly and with the kind of gentle efficiency Lee had to admire. If anyone could pull him through, these people could.

She had lost track of time when Sister returned to find her huddled in the chair, biting back tears of frustration and anger that it should have happened to someone she loved so much. Glancing from the patient to Lee's stricken face, Sister touched her gently on the shoulder and whispered, 'Why don't you go and get some fresh air, or a cup of coffee. It will do you good and there's really nothing you can do here, you know.'

Lee stared up at her as if scarcely aware of what she was saying, then she rose wearily to her feet. The night seemed endless.

'You're right, I'm not doing any good at all am I.' She brushed a hand through her hair. 'A cup of coffee sounds like a good idea, but you will call me . . . ?'

'Of course, although there hasn't been any change and we don't really anticipate one, not for several hours at least.'

'All the same,' Lee smiled, waveringly. 'I'll wait in the coffee lounge for a while if you don't mind. I don't want to leave, not yet. I know the first few hours can be crucial and I'd rather be here if . . .'

Sister's hand rested briefly over her own as they stood outside the door. 'He's fighting and that is important.' Sister Raymond couldn't have been more than twenty-five but she spoke as if to someone much younger and with the quiet authority which had made her popular throughout the hospital and particularly on her own ward.

Lee nodded bleakly. 'You're very kind.' She moved away, scarcely knowing where she was going, knowing she mustn't take up the staff's time and yet wishing desperately there was someone she could talk to.

The coffee machine gave out a plastic beaker of watery brown liquid which tasted like an odd mixture between coffee and chocolate but she sipped at it without even noticing. Her hands were shaking as she sank into one of the large, comfortable chairs and stared at the clock. Four-thirty. Please God let him get through the night. She rested her head against her hand and closed her eyes.

Doors swished quietly open and closed. She didn't look up until the footsteps came towards her, then, thinking it must be Sister Raymond, she turned and rose unsteadily to her feet.

'Grant. Oh Grant, thank God.' Without realising it she was in his arms being held tightly and he was stroking her hair.

'It's all right,' he murmured. 'I'm here now.' Holding both her hands he led her back to the chair. 'What happened?' For the first time as he looked at her she saw the desperate lines of tiredness and tension in his face. 'I just got back from seeing a patient when the hospital called. It's Tom isn't it?'

She nodded, sinking into the chair, her head lowered. 'He had another heart attack. It's bad.'

'Oh my God.' He sank his face into his hands then dragged them slowly away and reached out for her. 'I must go and see him. Have you . . .'

'Yes, they let me sit with him for a while. Oh Grant, he looks so desperately ill. I couldn't bear it if he . . . if he . . .'

'Don't.' His voice rasped and with a quick movement he bent and kissed her. 'My poor darling, you've had a rotten time, but don't let's talk about anything except the fact that he's going to make it.'

'I want to believe it.' She brushed a hand over her eyes. 'I'm so glad you're here.'

He brushed the hair gently back from her face. 'Then do believe it.' He tried to laugh. 'Surely between us we must have some pull.'

'Let me come with you, please.' She was on her feet, swaying a little with tiredness. 'Please Grant. I can bear it if you're with me.'

He studied her, grimly. 'You needn't worry that I shall ever leave you again.' He paused, then nodded. 'Okay, as long as you promise not to pass out on me, not yet at least.'

'I promise.'

It was comforting to have his arm around her. Somewhere it registered vaguely in her brain that he hadn't been out with Christy after all.

They had just walked through the swings doors when Sister Raymond came towards them. Lee felt her heart miss a beat and instinctively Grant's arm tightened round her.

'Bear up,' he murmured, gruffly, but she could see the sudden tightening of his own mouth as he hurried her along the corridor, the sound of their footsteps echoing in the night stillness.

'Oh Dr Sinclair, they managed to contact you then, I'm so glad.' Anne Raymond smiled her recognition. 'I was just coming to find Dr Forrester.'

Lee felt her knees buckle and would have fallen if Grant hadn't held her. 'It's not . . .' She couldn't bring herself to say it and was aware of Grant's white face above her own.

Incredibly, Sister smiled. 'No, Doctor, he's fine.'

'Oh thank God.' She closed her eyes and felt some of the tension slip out of Grant's hold upon her.

'Has there been any change, any change at all?' he asked.

'That's why I came to find you. Yes, there has, it's very slight of course, but he is definitely breathing more easily and is sleeping quite peacefully now. In fact I was going to suggest that it might be a good idea if you were to go home for a few hours and get some rest. I promise we will call you if there is any change, but I think he's going to be all right.' She looked at them both. 'I probably shouldn't say it but we get an instinct about these things and I know it sounds silly, but we're usually right.'

'I know what you mean.' Grant looked at Lee. She knew her face was colourless and her eyes felt raw from the lack of sleep but she was past caring. The only thing that mattered was that he was here. 'Thank you, Sister, we'll take your advice, for a few hours at least.' He drew Lee's coat gently round her shoulders as Sister hurried away. His hands turned the collar up, holding it against her face. 'Come on, I'm going to take you home.'

She felt too drained to ask where 'home' was. She sat in the car feeling the tiredness wash over her, there was a sense of elation too. She was glad when he made no attempt to start the engine and they just sat in the semi-darkness.

'He really is going to be all right, isn't he?'

'Do you doubt it?'

She turned to look at him and shook her head. 'No, somehow I don't, not now. But I was so afraid. I didn't know how I'd face it without you.' She buried her face in her hands but suddenly she was in his arms again and he was kissing her fiercely, possessively, as if to shut out all the doubts.

'Darling,' his voice was gruff as he released her, momentarily. 'If you only knew how I felt when I got that call and realised you were here alone. I drove like a maniac and when I saw you just sitting there, looking so lost, I thought . . . Oh my God, I thought.' His hands gripped her shoulders. 'I love you, you know that, don't you?'

Her answer was muffled by yet another kiss. She

could scarcely believe what was happening. Perhaps even now it was all part of the nightmare and when she opened her eyes he would have vanished. Her hands held him away.

'But what about Christy?' The words were torn from her in desperation. 'You're going to marry her. How can you love me?'

He was staring at her, incredulously. 'Christy? Are you serious? For heaven's sake how does she come into this?'

'But . . . but I thought . . . I heard you talking . . . about marriage.'

She heard his swift mutter of impatience. 'My dear girl, if you had listened to the entire conversation instead of running away, you might have realised that it wasn't Christy I intended to marry, but you.'

'Me?' Her eyes widened.

'Well who else?'

'But I thought . . .'

'Yes, I realise now what you must have thought and I could kick myself for not going after you and making you listen, but the truth is that after Beth died I really thought I would never want to think about marriage again. It was Christy who made me realise what a fool I was, that I was running the risk of losing you because of it.'

Lee stared at him. 'She said that?'

He laughed softly at her look of amazement then became serious. 'Christy happens to be Beth's sister, my love. Since Beth died she has kept me sane, gradually taught me that life doesn't stop just because someone you love happens to die, and I realise now that she was right.'

She couldn't speak. It was all too much to take in.

'But what about you and Charles?'

'Charles,' she laughed, almost hysterically. 'Oh yes, Charles.'

'He asked you to marry him.'

'And I said no.' Her hands touched his face, teased the hair at the nape of his neck and she heard him moan softly before he gathered her up fiercely in his arms. 'I had to say no. I could only spend the rest of my life with someone I love, with you, my darling, if you want me.'

His answer was a kiss which seemed to go on for ever, and which left her in no doubt at all what the answer would be.

Doctor Nurse Romances

Romance in modern medical life

Read more about the lives and loves of doctors and nurses in the fascinatingly different backgrounds of contemporary medicine. These are the four Doctor Nurse romances to look out for next month.

AUSTRIAN INTERLUDE
Lee Stafford

SECOND CHANCE AT LOVE
Zara Holman

TRIO OF DOCTORS
Lindsay Hicks

CASSANDRA BY CHANCE
Betty Neels

Buy them from your usual paperback stockist, or write to: Mills & Boon Reader Service, P.O. Box 236, Thornton Rd, Croydon, Surrey CR9 3RU, England. Readers in South Africa-write to: Mills & Boon Reader Service of Southern Africa, Private Bag X3010, Randburg, 2125.

Mills & Boon
the rose of romance

Doctor Nurse Romances

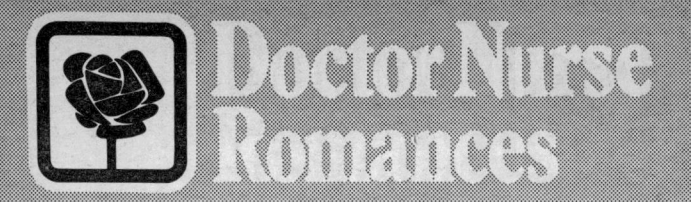

Amongst the intense emotional pressures of modern medical life, doctors and nurses often find romance. Read about their lives and loves in the other three Doctor Nurse titles available this month.

NURSE OVERBOARD
by Meg Wisgate

Nurse Kate Trelawney is enjoying her private nursing assignment at a villa on the beautiful Greek island of Corfu, until the presence of the supercilious French doctor Laurent de Kerouac threatens to cast a cloud over her Mediterranean idyll . . .

WRONG DOCTOR JOHN
by Kate Starr

At first dismayed when she is transferred to the unattractive Eye Clinic attached to Sydney's Southern Cross Hospital, Nurse Emma Brown soon finds how mistaken her opinion has been. Is she equally mistaken about young Doctor John Harding?

EMERGENCY NURSE
by Grace Read

Staff Nurse Laurel Swann – nicknamed Laurel the Unflappable – finds it hard to live up to her name after she has met Bruce Tyson, the dynamic surgeon in the Accident and Emergency Department.

Mills & Boon
the rose of romance

How to join in a whole new world of romance

It's very easy to subscribe to the Mills & Boon Reader Service. As a regular reader, you can enjoy a whole range of special benefits. Bargain offers. Big cash savings. Your own free Reader Service newsletter, packed with knitting patterns, recipes, competitions, and exclusive book offers.

We send you the very latest titles each month, postage and packing free – no hidden extra charges. There's absolutely no commitment – you receive books for only as long as you want.

We'll send you details. Simply send the coupon – or drop us a line for details about the Mills & Boon Reader Service Subscription Scheme.

Post to: Mills & Boon Reader Service, P.O. Box 236, Thornton Road, Croydon, Surrey CR9 3RU, England.

*Please note: READERS IN SOUTH AFRICA please write to: Mills & Boon Reader Service of Southern Africa, Private Bag X3010, Randburg 2125, S. Africa.

Please send me details of the Mills & Boon Subscription Scheme.

NAME (Mrs/Miss) _____ EP3

ADDRESS _____

COUNTY/COUNTRY _____ POST/ZIP CODE _____

BLOCK LETTERS, PLEASE

Mills & Boon
the rose of romance